MAKE
YOURSELF
BETTER

*A Practical Guide to Restoring Your Body's
Wellbeing through Ancient Medicine*

Philip Weeks

SINGING
DRAGON

LONDON AND PHILADELPHIA

First published in 2012
by Singing Dragon
an imprint of Jessica Kingsley Publishers
116 Pentonville Road
London N1 9JB, UK
and
400 Market Street, Suite 400
Philadelphia, PA 19106, USA

www.singingdragon.com

Copyright © Philip Weeks 2012
Illustrations copyright © Chloe Douglass 2012

Library of Congress Cataloging in Publication Data
A CIP catalog record for this book is available from the Library of Congress

British Library Cataloguing in Publication Data
A CIP catalogue record for this book is available from the British Library

ISBN 978 1 84819 012 2
eISBN 978 0 85701 077 3

Printed and bound in Great Britain

CONTENTS

ACKNOWLEDGEMENTS

I wrote this book with a lot of help and support.

First, my inspiration in natural medicine was initially ignited by Richard Schulze and Kitty Campion. Also, the many teachers on the way: the late John Morley, Stephen Macallan, Christopher Hobbs, John and Angela Hicks, Peter Mole, Lillian Bridges, Danielle Lo Rito and Salim Khan. My mother and father for encouraging me on my path in natural medicine. Gomati for her help in the initial stages of this project. Linda Day for her unending support. Arjuna and Purnamasi, Andrew Mason, Rosemary Wilson, Sara and Howard, and Chloe Douglass for her wonderful illustrations.

Veda and our son Dhanvantari.

Jessica Kingsley for her unfaltering belief and unrelenting encouragement.

Last, I dedicate this work to my patients who ultimately are the best teachers for me.

DISCLAIMER

If you decide to make any lifestyle changes or undertake a cleanse/detox routine, you will first need to consult a medical doctor and/or a suitably qualified practitioner. They will assess whether any of the changes or routines are suitable for you by considering your current state of health and pre-existing conditions, as well as any medication you may be taking or have taken in the past.

Many foods, herbs and spices can occasionally cause allergic reactions. Any of the recommendations in this book could be potentially dangerous, even deadly, especially if you are already ill or suffer from a disease.

Every effort has been made to ensure that the information contained in this book is correct, but it should not in any way be substituted for medical advice. Readers should always consult a qualified medical practitioner before incorporating any of the therapies mentioned in this book into their treatment plan, whether conventional, complementary or alternative. Neither the author nor the publisher takes any responsibility for the consequences of any decision made as a result of the information contained in this book.

THE WHEEL OF HEALTH

Patients often ask me how and why a particular health problem has descended upon them. Quite naturally, they are keen for its unwanted presence to disappear so they can return to a 'normal' lifestyle.

With some trepidation I explain that their normal lifestyle may well have contributed to the emergence of their condition. I try to help them understand that by removing unwelcome symptoms and listening to their body's pleas, opportunities will arise for them to improve their health.

Many of the world's oldest healing systems have wonderful analogies about how and why we become unwell. Reading about daily life thousands of years ago, it's amazing to see how little our needs have changed and how, even now, even with knowledge and accumulated wisdom, we still dive headlong into the man-traps of life.

Of course, our physical worlds look quite different, but our basic motivation – to remain happy – remains. We are all driven by the desire to achieve something while at the same time remaining comfortable and content.

The world we live in is changing more quickly than ever. Looking back just 5, 10 or 15 years we can see how technology is changing the way we live our lives in a short amount of time. The way this impacts our lives is very mixed. We can get what we want quicker, communication is instantaneous. Technology has given us huge benefits, but it has its price. The pace of change is faster than most of us can keep up with.

The concepts in this book are not new, but are a synergy of my study of ancient medical techniques from India, China and Greece and more recent understandings of heath and disease. These concepts have developed from my work with thousands of patients over the last 12 years and with what works in clinical practice. In this book I have drawn on some of this ancient wisdom and placed it into a modern framework to make its application as practical as possible. What I hope you will do is try to adopt some of the basic principles of these historical doctrines and integrate them into your daily patterns and routines. I believe that ancient cultures have a treasure trove of important accumulated wisdom that we now need, more than ever before, not as a replacement for modern science but as an important companion.

I have used the term 'the wheel of health' as it seems to be a universal concept that what goes around comes around. Just like a wheel turning, everything we encounter has some effect upon our life journey.

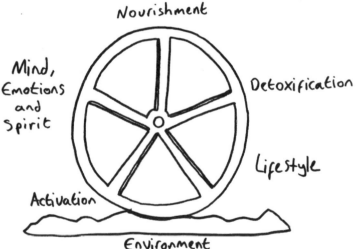

The body we have been given is a result of not just the genetics from our parents, but also the environment and conditions that were present when we were formed in the womb. I have represented this as the wheel itself. It is understood from ancient medicine that some people are born with a more robust 'wheel' than others. This makes sense as some people can essentially abuse their body for years and years and live to a ripe old age, whereas others have to really look after themselves just to get by. It is important to consider our constitution as we need to make sure our lifestyle and all of the other areas are in balance and in harmony with it. We are all different – we need to find out what works for us.

Every moment we are alive we interface with our environment. The era we live in, the place we live in, the people we live with are represented by the road the wheel is turning on. Although we have a somewhat limited choice as to the environment we live in, there is no discounting the impact it has on our wellbeing. Being conscious and aware of our individual needs can help to empower us to make healthy choices as to our surroundings, the people with whom we share our lives and even the substances we apply to our body and surround ourselves with. What road we choose determines the rate at which wear and tear erodes the rims and spokes of our wheel: a smooth, even path, for example, creates little stress while a sharp incline and bumpy terrain places greater stress upon the whole structure.

The wheel has five imaginary spokes, providing a buffer zone between the wildly spinning rim and the slow-turning hub. The keys to the wheel of health are these spokes. The spokes represent our body's integrated and self-regulatory rules of engagement. So, as with spokes on a physical wheel, keeping those on our wheel of health in a state of balance and equilibrium is the secret to a smooth journey through life. Each spoke represents a factor that affects the health of our being right now.

The first spoke of the wheel represents *nourishment*. This is what we put into our body in the form of air, liquid and food.

This is the first spoke of the wheel as it is completely fundamental to our wellbeing. Nutrition is probably the single most important consideration that creates health or disease. Although nutrition is a vast subject I believe there to be some basic principles that if we adhere to can help us enjoy better health.

The second spoke of the wheel is *detoxification*. Nourishment is essential, but without good detoxification and elimination we will become contaminated by our own wastes and overwhelmed by external environmental poisons, resulting in sickness and disease. Encouraging good elimination helps the body work better and I believe is essential when combating disease. I will discuss ways to encourage healthy detoxification through our elimination organs: the bowels, kidneys, liver and skin.

The third spoke is our *lifestyle*. This is the way we live our life, our daily routine. When we get up, when we go to sleep. When we eat, where we eat. This spoke also relates to the amount of rest we take.

The fourth spoke is *activation*: what we do to move our body, exercise and activity.

The fifth spoke is our *mind, emotions and spirit*. This is in some ways the most important but yet the most challenging to transform. How we think, what we feel. It is our connection with ourselves, the universe, the divine.

And finally, the centre of the wheel – the balance of everything. The hub of our imaginary wheel represents the calm of the storm, a focal point from where we find that nothing is too much trouble and from where we function with peak efficiency, energy, ease and joy.

The more we move away from our idealised centre the more we feel the effects of inertia or chaos. Consequently, the greater outward force pulls us ever closer to the rim, ultimately placing us between the bumpy terrain and the rim itself. This is a difficult place to be – and not an easy one to regain a more stable position from. My aim with this book, as it is with my patients, is through supporting all aspects of the wheel to come to a place of optimal wellbeing.

Chapter 1

OUR ENVIRONMENT

Our environment has a huge amount of influence on our health and wellbeing. From temperature, humidity, quality of sanitation, altitude…so many different factors. Human beings are incredibly versatile and adaptive even in extremes and are able to find strategies to adapt and survive in all kinds of environments.

The World Health Organization has estimated that 24 per cent of the global disease burden and 23 per cent of all deaths can be attributed to environmental factors (Prüss-Üstün and Corvalán 2006). The biggest killer in the developing world is still a lack of clean water.

Ancient medical texts talk about the importance of living in an environment conducive to good health and wellbeing.

Arguably the most profound development in health care in the nineteenth and twentieth centuries happened after the discovery of bacteria. Through this came an understanding of the importance of good sanitation, drinking clean water and eating uncontaminated food. These principles are not new – the ancient Romans and Greeks had an understanding that sanitation was a basic principle for a healthy life. However, during the nineteenth and twentieth centuries the impact of allowing people access to clean water, a regular supply of food and good sanitation has arguably been the main contributor to the extension in people's lives today.

Conversely, in the twentieth century environmental factors have come into being which as humans we have never experienced or been exposed to in all of the millions of years we have been on the planet – man-made chemicals, contraceptives in our water supply (Wu *et al.* 2009), plastics and pesticides in our food chain, electromagnetic and radioactive radiation.

There are numerous areas to explore in regard to these and their role in human health. I believe that these influences, along with a degrading quality of nutrition, are now manifesting in our health, both as a race and as individuals. Cancer, type II diabetes and obesity are becoming commonplace, as is the proliferation of chronic and degenerative conditions.

There are factors that feature frequently in my clinic that I would like to explore with you. Some of these environmental factors accumulate in our body, either from exposure, or because they are deliberately placed into the body. The result is disease and fatigue.

EXOGENOUS (EXTERNAL) TOXINS

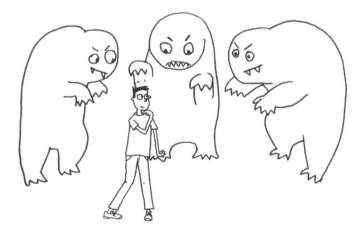

Outside our body is a world full of substances that we have to come to terms with, many of which exist in our own homes, gardens and workplaces. Many are naturally occurring – tetanus, botulism and toxic metals such as arsenic and lead are examples of naturally occurring toxins. However, many more are man-made, which in our genetic history we have never been exposed to before. And the list of substances to which we are being exposed to – in some cases voluntarily – is growing all the time. In a typical day, we could be exposing ourselves to, or ingesting:

- artificial colourings, preservatives and E numbers

- cleaning sprays

- dioxin

- fluoride

- formaldehyde

- hair dye

- heavy metals

- herbicides

- perfumes, deodorants

- pesticides

- phthalates (often listed as fragrance on packaging)

- parabens

- tobacco smoke

- weed killers

- xenoestrogens

- volatile organic compounds.

The problem with many of these chemicals and substances is that they are persistent and can linger in the environment for many years. They also tend to accumulate in animals and humans. This process is called *bio-accumulation* and occurs because the chemicals are attracted to fatty tissues. Although many of these are quite probably harmless, we know many that are definitely not.

PLASTICS

This subject deserves a bit of an explanation, especially as most of us are exposed to plastics in our daily life.

There are two substances to get to grips with if we want to understand the way plastics can undermine our health: bisophenol A and phthalates.

Bisophenol A (BPA) is a chemical used to harden plastic, typically present in the inside of tinned food, baby's bottles and plastic containers. First created in 1891, it has been known to mimic oestrogen since the 1930s.

The problem is that it isn't stable and leaches into food and liquids. With it comes all kind of negative health effects. It is suspected to be the reason sperm counts are declining and worldwide hormone-related cancers are on the increase.

To give an idea of how pervasive this substance is you only have to read about a study of pregnant women in 2011, which discovered that 96 per cent of those tested had traces of BPA in their body (Woodruff, Zota and Schwartz 2011).

Phthalates are also present in many plastics, and are used to improve their pliability and flexibility. They are present in toys, plastic containers, vinyl flooring – the list is endless.

Once again they are a potent hormone disrupter. In my clinic I see girls as young as six years old who are now going into puberty. Studies have made the link between exposure to this compound and early puberty in girls (Foodconsumer 2010). Phthalates are oestrogenic and can contribute to insulin resistance and therefore make us more likely to be fat (Stahlhut *et al.* 2007).

Plastics, pesticides and a number of other man-made chemicals are known to be not only carcinogenic but also disruptive to hormones, which is why they are also referred to as 'gender benders'. Gender benders are believed to be responsible for the higher female child populations among Arctic tribes. In Greenland and eastern Russia, girls outnumber boys by two to one.

I believe also that exposure to these chemicals could be contributing to the increase in cancer rates. Incidences of testicular cancer in the UK, for example, have been rising steadily since the 1940s.

This is also happening in many other European countries. In France, cancer in men has almost doubled (+93%) and has increased in women by 84 per cent over the past 25 years (European Trade Union Institute 2009). Only a small part of these increases can be attributed to population growth (25%) and ageing (20%).

So why is cancer on the rise? And why is the male population becoming less fertile? It seems to me it is something to do with our environment.

MERCURY

The toxins in your teeth

Mercury accounts for approximately half of a dental amalgam filling, and the mercury vapour released by amalgam fillings increases when we drink hot liquids and eat. There is evidence showing that the level of mercury in the brain tissue of foetuses, newborns and young children is directly proportional to the number of amalgam fillings the mother has (Drasch *et al.* 1994).

Mercury amalgam has been the subject of much controversy ever since it was first used in the nineteenth century. Mercury was first employed as a material in fillings because it has the ability to dissolve powders of other metals such as tin, copper, nickel and silver. Originally mixed with silver dust, mercury was first used as a dental material in 1830. Initial teething problems (pun unintended!) arose because it would expand excessively, often dislodging when the patient consumed hot food or drink.

Even after this problem was solved, mercury was well known for its toxic effects. In the nineteenth century it was prescribed as a medicine for syphilis, but dosage was always tricky – too high a dosage would result in fatal mercury poisoning. When mercury fillings were first introduced, dentists reported loss of motor control, fatigue and even symptoms of dementia in some patients.

Such was the outcry from the dentists that in 1845 the American Society of Dental Surgeons asked its members to sign a pledge never to use mercury again. However, from a dentist's point of view it was (and still is) an ideal material, being cheap, very durable and easy to install in the teeth. And, as the only alternative to the prohibitively expensive gold, the use of amalgam began to grow as the nineteenth century progressed.

In 1859 the American Society of Dental Surgeons disbanded and was replaced by the pro-amalgam American Dental Association. By 1900, mercury fillings were established as the standard in Europe and the rest of the world. However, in the 1920s the debate became active again. After noticing side-effects from using mercury in his laboratory, Professor Alfred E. Stock at the Kaiser Wilhelm Institute in Germany published a number of papers linking amalgam fillings with detrimental side-effects.

After more than 150 years, the mercury debate is still raging.

Mad as hatters

In the nineteenth century, milliners devised a complicated set of processes to transform animal fur into finished hats. A solution made from mercury enabled the fibres of the fur to mat together before a finishing process steamed the fur to shape and create the final top hat. This often took place in unventilated conditions, so hatters would continually inhale mercury vapour. Symptoms of mercury poisoning, including trembling, loss of coordination, slurred speech, memory loss, fatigue and personality change, became commonplace among those working in the industry. Thus was born 'mad hatter syndrome'. And though mercury is no longer used in hat-making, mad hatter syndrome is still very much with us.

While scientists agree that excessive exposure to mercury can cause serious health problems, it seems that they differ on the effects of moderate exposure.

Bodies representing the dental profession continually state that exposure to mercury from fillings is low. However, in 1998 the World Health Organization (WHO) declared that there is no safe level of exposure to mercury. Crematoriums in the UK have been given strict guidelines for reducing mercury pollution, which is caused when fillings are vaporised in the burning process. Crematoriums are predicted to be the biggest source of airborne mercury pollution by 2020.

Mercury is not rendered chemically inert in dental fillings. The amount absorbed from dental fillings exceeds toxic thresholds for mercury published by several governments. The US Environmental Protection Agency's reference dose for mercury, for example, is 3.84 micrograms/day, while Health Canada prescribes 1.4 micrograms/day as a tolerable daily intake. Yet a 1991 WHO report concluded that a person with one mercury filling will absorb between 3 and 17 micrograms of mercury per day. The consensus average estimate is around 10–12 micrograms absorbed per day and levels for some individuals may be as high as 100 micrograms/day. Many people are not aware that they are slowly and insidiously being poisoned by their fillings. Perhaps unsurprisingly then, many people suffering with apparently unrelated symptoms report health benefits after amalgam extraction.

I have a mouthful of mercury fillings – what do I do?

The more you chew, the more mercury is released into your body. This can be significant if you eat a lot of raw food. I have found, however, that wheatgrass – a cleanser par excellence – is great for pulling mercury out of the body. The downside is that wheatgrass can also take the mercury directly out of fillings. So, if you have amalgam fillings, drink wheatgrass through a straw until they've been replaced.

Mercury removal is a very delicate job that should be undertaken by a specialist mercury-free dentist. You'll need to be given a separate air supply during the process as 80 per cent of mercury vapour that you inhale goes into the bloodstream.

But the real work begins once the fillings have been removed. This is the time to clear the body of all the ingested mercury once and for all. I treat my patients with burdock, yellow dock and, depending on an individual's needs, sometimes homeopathic medicines. Coriander is an excellent mercury detoxifying medicine, known for its ability to pull mercury from brain tissue. Other measures such as colonics, the internal use of clay and saunas will encourage the body to excrete metals and restore the normal function of cells.

Warning: If you decide to have your amalgam fillings removed it is imperative that this is undertaken by an accomplished dentist who is familiar with how to remove them, and that they make every effort to keep your mercury exposure, particularly by vapour, to an absolute minimum. Fillings should be replaced gradually and carefully with bio-compatible composite fillings.

VACCINES

The safety and effectiveness of vaccination has been the subject of heated debate over the last ten years. I am asked almost daily about my view on vaccination and whether it is a good idea for someone to vaccinate their child, or themselves.

It is a complicated issue. One side of the debate states that vaccines are the only way to prevent dangerous disease; the other proclaims that they are ineffective, dangerous and amount to a potential medical time bomb.

The merits and demerits of either side of this dispute are far beyond the scope of this book. However, there are some interesting facts to consider. From 1911 to 1935, the four leading causes of childhood deaths from infectious diseases in the USA were diphtheria, pertussis (whooping cough), scarlet fever and measles. However, by 1945 the combined death rates from these causes had declined by 95 per cent, *before* the implementation of mass immunisation programmes (Buttram 2000). As the reduction in death rates from childhood diseases dropped before the implementation of mass vaccination, some medical researchers have concluded that this is actually due to the widespread improvements in sanitation and nutrition in the previous 100 years (Jeffreys 1999).

Vaccination efficacy aside, vaccines contain a surprising number of additives. Some of these additives have been found to increase IgE (immunoglobulin E) levels, which is the antibody present in those people with allergies (Tenpenny 2008). In a study of young people in Melbourne, Australia, those who had been fully immunised as children were found to be at higher risk of having asthma when they were adults (Benke *et al.* 2004).

What's in a vaccine?

Although there is academic dispute about the ability of vaccines to prevent disease, for me the main controversy lies in the cocktail of ingredients.

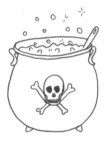

Vaccines contain surprising ingredients, some of which are listed below (Centre for Disease Control and Prevention 2010). Some of these ingredients are known toxins, which need to be metabolised and processed.

DTaP/IPV – diphtheria, tetanus, pertussis (whooping cough) and polio:

- aluminium hydroxide
- amino acids
- formaldehyde
- MRC-5 cellular protein
- neomycin sulphate

19

- 2-phenoxyethanol
- phosphate buffers
- polysorbate.

Influenza/flu:

- beta-propiolactone
- egg protein
- neomycin
- polymyxin B
- polyoxyethylene 9-10 nonyl phenol (Triton N-101, Octoxynol-9)
- thimerosal (mercury).

Polio:

- calf serum protein
- formaldehyde
- monkey kidney tissue
- neomycin
- 2-phenoxyethanol
- polymyxin B
- streptomycin.

MMR – measles, mumps and rubella:

- amino acid
- bovine albumin or serum
- chick embryo fibroblasts
- human serum albumin

- gelatin
- glutamate
- neomycin
- phosphate buffers
- sorbitol
- sucrose
- vitamins.

Personally, it seems to me like a witches' brew worthy of Macbeth. Each manufacturer has slightly different formulas, dependent on where and when the vaccines are made. The list of ingredients is usually available on the manufacturer's website.

Vaccination and natural medicine

I believe that whether we choose to vaccinate ourselves or our children, we need to be fully informed about the risks.

If you decide against vaccination, you'll need to know how to recognise and manage childhood diseases and when it's necessary for you or your child to see a health professional.

Children and vaccines

There are a number of approaches that can be applied to children who have not been vaccinated. Many people working in the alternative health arena, for example, encourage children to get childhood diseases such as measles, mumps and chicken pox. There is immunological research to support the idea that contracting and recovering from a childhood disease such as measles benefits the immune system. Some consider it an important part of exercising the immune system to prepare a child for adult life. Indeed, I know of several parents who have organised measles parties so their children can get infected and then be actively supported through the process.

I strongly believe that if children are carefully monitored and supported through their childhood diseases, they are less likely to get problems with allergies and autoimmune disorders as adults.

Warning: Whether you decide to vaccinate or not, both options carry risks to your health. You should get suitable personalised medical guidance before making your decision.

ELECTROMAGNETIC RADIATION

Many of us will have heard of the concerns regarding electro-magnetic fields or EMFs. This may have come from reports from individuals living near mobile phone masts with symptoms such as tiredness, depression, immune deficiencies and increased mental health issues – symptoms which subside when they reduce their exposure by moving house or by implementing EMF protection measures.

Dr George Carloa, a public health scientist, headed the first multi-million dollar research in 1993 to assess the safety of mobile phones. The programme was funded by the cell phone industry. Over a period of six years, his research made very alarming discoveries linking mobile/cellular phones to serious health problems and diseases. On submitting his findings to the industry, he was discredited and his research ignored by the very people who paid him to carry it out. He and other researchers came to certain conclusions regarding how EMFs cause damage:

- Radiation from mobile phones penetrates deep into the brains of developing children

- Radiation from mobile phones break down the blood-brain barrier, leaving the brain more vulnerable to damage from environmental toxins

(Carlo and Schram 2001)

The effect of electromagnetic radiation is controversial and there are studies on either side with some suggesting that EMF exposure is dangerous and others suggesting it is safe. The problem is that EMFs are a new phenomenon – as a species we have never been exposed to them before. I think exposure should be classified as a potential form of stress, and as an influence that can interfere with health and cellular communication, and a possible cause of free radicals.

I think it is prudent to protect our children by avoiding mobile phone use, and for us to minimise exposure as much as possible:

- Don't keep your mobile phone in your pocket or next to your body all day. Men should be particularly aware of the potential effect on fertility.

- Avoid using cordless phones and use a regular wired analogue one.

- If you choose to have Wi-Fi in your home, at least disable it when not in use.

- Better still, have a wired internet connection with a special dLAN adaptor which will turn your home's circuitry into an extension to your computer network, allowing you to access the web from any electrical socket in your house.

- Avoid obvious EMF exposure such as electricity substations, overhead pylons and microwave ovens (either in the house or food cooked with them).

- Some EMF exposure is unavoidable, but at least ensure that your sleeping area is as free of it as possible. Electric alarm clocks can sometimes emit very high EMFs. Avoid using your mobile phone as an alarm clock or having it in your bedroom at night, and avoid having a TV in your bedroom. Choose a wooden bed frame and a non-spring mattress. Metal can act like an antenna amplifying the intensity of electromagnetic fields. Avoid electric blankets.

TESTING FOR TOXINS

In my clinic I have had the opportunity to test thousands of people for the presence of environmental toxins. I have been interested in discovering what is stuck deep in the body with a view to understanding the cause of the illness. Once an unwanted substance is discovered and identified then at least it gives us an opportunity to encourage its removal from the body.

The normal biochemistry tests from a doctor or hospital will assess factors such as levels of iron, kidney and liver function, number of red and white blood cells, blood sugar levels and others. These tests are certainly necessary for ruling out major pathology or disease processes and will reveal, for example, if someone is suffering from an infection.

Routine blood tests, though, do not assess levels of toxins or of trace elements present in an individual. What we need to know is why the body has created this disease. Is it from malnutrition, such as a lack of trace elements? Is it because of a toxicity burden? If so, which toxins are they? There are a number of methods of assessing the bio-accumulation in an individual:

- *Fat biopsy.* This is where a needle takes a sample of fat cells which is then tested for the presence of chemicals, especially pesticides.

- *Hair analysis.* Here, a sample of hair is taken and analysed, as this form of analysis shows what the body is excreting as well as the balance of minerals. This can be useful in determining the presence of toxic minerals such as heavy metals like cadmium and mercury.

- *Bio-resonance testing.* This is a method of testing for certain frequencies present in the body, which can give a clue as to what might be contaminating an individual. This is carried out using a bio-feedback mechanism such as the Vega machine. The accuracy of this is somewhat dependent on the skill of the machine operator, although when carried out competently it can be very helpful in toxin identification. If something is discovered with this method I will often use another test to confirm the results.

- *DNA adducts.* This is a more recent test created by a biochemist, Dr John McLaren Howard. I have found this extremely useful. Toxins may be present in an individual such as in the fat, organs and cell membranes. However, the most dangerous ones can be those that are actually stuck to the DNA, called DNA adducts. The effects are incredibly insidious as the toxin or adduct can affect the DNA structure and shape as well as interfering with DNA replication and repair. The toxin can affect the way a gene expresses itself. As you can imagine, this can have huge and devastating repercussions in the way the body functions and repairs itself. I almost always discover DNA adducts present in people with cancer and those with neurological diseases such as Parkinson's disease, as well as those with unexplained symptoms that don't fit into a category and who are often labelled as having 'chronic fatigue'.

Just going through some of the tests carried out on my patients in the last few months reveals the kind of toxins typically present in many people, as shown in Table 1.1.

Table 1.1 Some of the most commonly discovered
toxins detected in blood samples

Toxin	Source
Lindane	Pesticide and insecticide, also a wood preservative. It is still used in the treatment of scabies.
DDT	The first synthetic pesticide, but now restricted because of its toxicity, although still used in the developing world.
Hair dye	This can contain a number of toxic components, although I frequently find p-Phenylenediamine.
Mercury	Amalgam 'silver' fillings are usually the source, but also some environmental sources such as energy-saving light bulbs and in vaccinations.
Formaldehyde	Used in wood composites such as MDF, chipboard and plywood.
Nitrosamines	Present in tobacco smoke, beer, some insecticides and processed meat, especially bacon.
Pentachlorophenol	Once widely used as a wood preservative, this has mostly been banned because of its toxicity.
Aluminium	Found in some pots and pans and teapots, cooking foil and as a preservative in vaccinations.

DETOX TO GET WELL

In my experience, improving people's ability to detoxify greatly increases their ability to get well.

Although the body is fully equipped to deal with its own metabolic toxins, it now has to confront many man-made substances that we were never designed to deal with. In Chapter 5, I discuss some of the ways we can encourage the body to process and eliminate toxins.

STEPS TO TAKE TO MINIMISE TOXINS AND THE EFFECTS OF ENVIRONMENTAL FACTORS

Plastics:

- Avoid cling film and plastic containers where possible.

- Use bisophenol A-free sports bottles and feeding bottles and beakers.

- Avoid non-stick frying pans; use iron or the new non-stick ceramic pans.

- Purchase water in glass bottles.

Toxic metals:

- Don't use aluminium pans; use glass, stainless steel or iron.

- Avoid mercury and all metals in your mouth.

Electromagnetic pollution:

- Keep your use of your mobile phone to a minimum.

- Don't have the mobile phone in the bedroom at night, or at least keep it a few feet away from the bed.

- Avoid electric blankets and electric alarm clocks.

Household:

- Use biodegradable eco-cleaners. If you need a stronger substance use bleach – although be aware that the fumes are toxic, but it will biodegrade.

- Use essential oils instead of synthetic air fresheners.

- New carpets and furniture release chemicals such as formaldehyde into the atmosphere – use plants to soak up the fumes.

- Adopt the Eastern practice of removing your shoes when entering the house – it helps to reduce physical and vibrational contamination.

Clothing:

- Avoid wearing clothes made from petrochemicals and instead wear cotton, wool and silk.
- Use biodegradable cleaners.
- Avoid chemicals used in dry cleaning – take clothes out of the plastic and let the chemicals out.

Cosmetics and personal hygiene:

- Use one of the many alternatives to toothpaste containing fluoride.
- Avoid tampons and sanitary towels that are bleached – instead use dioxin-free varieties or a menstrual cup.
- Choose natural alternatives over chemical cosmetics.
- Never use toxic head lice applications that contain insecticides. Use a lice comb and essential oils such as rosemary and neem.

Garden:

- Never use pesticides or insecticides to control insects, infestations or weeds. It is worth exploring other methods such as permaculture.

Pets:

- Many patients are able to trace back the trigger of their illness to being exposed to flea spray or powder. Avoid insecticides at all costs – try natural alternatives.

Chapter 2

OUR INTAKE

NUTRITION

When writing this chapter I decided to go to my local bookshop and explore what was available on the subject of nutrition. I wasn't the only one. There were a few other people there too. And they all had a similar look on their face…one of utter confusion. This seemed to be because the majority of books in this section were preoccupied with the current trend – weight loss. Themes included *The Atkins Diet Rediscovered*, *Eat Right for your Blood Type*, *Low GI*, or the comical *Skinny Bitch Diet*. In the field of nutrition, the title list is almost endless. People with conditions such as arthritis, skin complaints and even Alzheimer's were also well catered for in terms of dietary advice, but far less common were books on general nutrition.

OUR DIET HAS CHANGED

Over the last hundred years the way that food is grown, produced, processed and eaten has had a profound effect on people's diets worldwide. The West, for example, has seen a revolution in modern agricultural methods. Before the 1950s most food was grown organically, although the concept of using substances to control infestation is not new. Pyrethrum is a good example: an extract from the chrysanthemum genus, it was discovered in China and used to kill insects. It was adopted in Europe as early as the Napoleonic Wars in powder form as an insect repellent for soldiers.

Minerals such as sulphur were also used to control insects and mould growth, while fertilisers were predominantly made from animal and human sewage. This meant that nutrients would go back into the soil and remineralise the produce.

All this began to change around World War II with the advent of chemical pesticides, fertilisers, herbicides and fungicides. The thinking at this time was that crops required a minimal number of key ingredients to produce healthy food, principally nitrogen (N), phosphorus (P) and potassium (K).

This combination, known as NPK, allowed food growers to create a synthetic fertiliser which, initially, appeared to produce healthy crops and plants. What followed was a food revolution in the twentieth century – high yield crops, cheaper food and lower labour costs.

But...

Food produced using synthetic fertilisers and pesticides tends to be of poor nutritional content. In other words, it's not very good for you. Nitrogen, for instance, reduces the eventual levels of vitamin C in produce, while potassium reduces the plant's uptake of magnesium and phosphorus.

Furthermore, this simplified form of fertilisation fails to restock the soil with all of the minerals that the plants – and ultimately we – need. This results in the rapid depletion of the trace elements in the soil and in turn its overall chemistry.

Even with the minerals in the soil, there is no guarantee that they will be absorbed by the plant. Absorption is only possible if the right kind of fungus called the mycorrhiza – which means fungal roots – is present. Mycorrhiza serves as an interface between healthy soil and the plant roots. Mycorrhiza-assisted plants and crops are more likely to grow healthily. They will also be rich in nutrients. Modern agricultural methods that include the use of chemical fertilisers, pesticides and fungicides destroy mycorrhiza.

Many pesticides also act as chelating agents. Deriving from the Latin word for 'claw', chelating agents attach themselves to minerals and pull them from the soil. So as well as producing insufficiently nutritious food, insecticides, pesticides and fertilisers further deplete the soil. This massive demineralisation of our food, therefore, leads to the demineralisation of our body.

> NPK formulas, as legislated and enforced by State Departments of Agriculture, mean malnutrition, attack by insects, bacteria and fungi, weed takeover, crop loss in dry weather, and general loss of mental acuity in the population, leading to degenerative metabolic disease and early death. (Dr William A. Albrecht, a prolific researcher and writer on the effects of soil on health from 1918 to 1970, quoted in Clark 2007)

MONOCULTURE

Monoculture is the term used to describe the practice of growing a single crop, such as wheat or corn, in a given field, year after year. Because it maximises land use, reduces the need for labour and increases profits, it's easy to see why major commercial farmers are monoculture enthusiasts.

Nature, however, is not. Look at any field in the UK that has been left to its own devices. Before long you'll see hundreds of diverse plant species, wild flowers, grasses and insects appearing. Nature likes diversity and monoculture is the antithesis of this. Monoculture makes crops more prone to disease, pulls the nutrients out of the soil and increases the need for fertilisers and pesticides.

We can see that there has been a trend since the advent of industrialised and intensive farming. There has been an emphasis on macronutrients, such as protein, carbohydrate and fat, while the important micronutrients such as vitamins and minerals have declined.

SO HAVE ALL THESE CHANGES MADE ANY DIFFERENCE?

We can track the decline in nutrient content by analysing data published in HM Government's Composition of Foods documents, which are released periodically. In this example you can see how the once mineral-rich carrot has diminished in nutrient content since 1940.

Table 2.1 Carrots: An example of the decline in food mineral content in the last 60 years

Mineral	1940	2002	Reduction in nutrients
Calcium (Ca)	48.00	25.00	48% ⇓
Magnesium (Mg)	12.00	3.00	75% ⇓
Iron (Fe)	0.56	0.30	46% ⇓
Copper (Cu)	0.08	0.02	75% ⇓
Sodium (Na)	95.00	25.00	74% ⇓
Potassium (K)	224.00	170.00	24% ⇓
Phosphorus (P)	21.00	15.00	33% ⇓

Values shown in mg per 100g
Source: Thomas 2003

And it's not just the carrot that has suffered the indignity. Various researchers have discovered similar levels of vitamin and mineral reduction in a wide range of foods worldwide. Between 1940 and 1991, vegetables consumed in the UK lost significant levels of nutrients. On average, at the end of this 51-year period, our vegetables contained:

46 per cent less calcium

24 per cent less magnesium

27 per cent less iron

76 per cent less copper

49 per cent less sodium

16 per cent less potassium.

(Thomas 2003)

I believe these findings have serious implications for our health. And to make matters worse, our food is also being exposed to toxic chemicals.

PESTICIDES

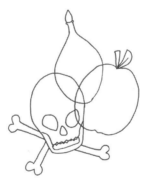

Chemical pesticides have changed our planet and our food beyond recognition. By 2007, over 1 billion tons of pesticides (Office of Pesticide Programs 2007) and 5 million tons of chemical fertilisers (Worthington 2001) were being used in the USA alone. And while they are mainly used in food production worldwide, 16 per cent of the world's pesticides are used on cotton (EJF 2007).

Life span of people who work with pesticides

I don't want to dwell too long on pesticides as the topic is too big to cover in this book. However, I frequently discover their presence in my patients, some of whom have never lived in the countryside. Often I find pesticides in the blood, and – more disturbingly – attached to a patient's DNA.

Some pesticides, such as DDT, take up to 30 years to biodegrade. Banned for use in agriculture in 1972 because of its immense toxicity, DDT is still used to kill mosquitoes in the developing world. DDT is carcinogenic and acts like an oestrogen in the body. Unfortunately DDT is present in most of us.

In France pesticides were found to be a contributing factor in brain tumours among vineyard workers. We also know that pesticide use increases the likelihood of neurological diseases and cancer and causes many additional, unknown effects.

According to the Stockholm Convention on Persistent Organic Pollutants, out of the top 12 most dangerous chemicals known to man, nine of them are pesticides (Stockholm Convention 2011).

IF YOU WANT TO BE HEALTHIER, EAT ORGANIC FOOD

In order to produce organically, we have to work with nature. It is the only way to produce crops with a consistently good yield and keep disease to a minimum. Organic food production methods include:

- *Crop rotation.* The way farming used to be. Crop rotation stops the soil from becoming depleted and protects it from pests and diseases. It relies on growing a number of different crops each year, such as potatoes, oats, peas or rye, then leaving the plot fallow for a year, before repeating the cycle.

- *Nourishing the soil.* Ways to nourish soil include growing 'green manure' – nurturing plants for the purpose of ploughing them back into the land – and the use of compost or manure. Compost and manure normally come from both plants and animals.

- *Biodynamic farming methods.* Here, farmers work with the phases of the moon and use homeopathic remedies. The nutritional bio-availability of the resulting produce seems to be even higher than in organically grown food.

Antioxidants are a key part of preventing a multitude of illnesses such as cancer, cardiovascular disease and other degenerative disorders. Organically produced fruit and vegetables have a greater concentration of antioxidants than conventionally grown produce (Woese *et al.* 1997).

Woese *et al.*'s study reviewed 150 research projects comparing organic and non-organic food, and concluded that organic foods have a trend towards fewer undesirable contaminants and higher desirable components (such as vitamins) compared to non-organic foods. Further studies have shown that:

- organic produce has significantly lower levels of pesticide and toxic residues (Baker *et al.* 2002)

- organic plant-based produce is nutritionally superior to non-organic food and on average has 25 per cent more nutrient content (Benbrook *et al.* 2008)

- organic milk contains more antioxidants and vitamins than non-organic milk. Studies have shown that on average it contains 63 per cent more omega 3 fatty acids and 50 per cent more vitamin E, and is 75 per cent higher in beta-carotene than conventionally produced milk (Butler *et al.* 2008; Ellis *et al.* 2006).

As long as agro-chemicals exist there will always be controversy about their effects and, to further vex the issue, we are also being exposed to the as yet unknown effects of genetically modified (GM) foods.

FOOD – MEDICINE – POISON

In many ancient cultures, substances that we ingest would be classified according to their effects on the body. They would fall into one or more of three categories:

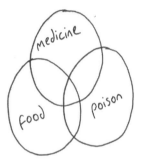

- *Food.* We consume food and assimilate its various components, which help give the body the substance to replenish, restore and rebuild. Food provides fuel for the body and gives it the base ingredients for us to replace tissues.

- *Medicine.* Medicine changes the way our body functions, such as its physiology or its actions, or provides something that is missing. Let's look at diuretics, for example. If the body has problems processing and excreting excess fluid, resulting in oedema, a diuretic would encourage the excretion of that fluid, thus helping to restore the system. A medicine may also act as a rejuvenator or a killer of pathogens.

- *Poison.* Poison undermines the correct and healthy homeostasis of the body. It disrupts the functioning of a cell or organ system, either subtly or radically, to a point that could ultimately kill us. One example is cyanide. It quickly poisons the body by affecting the heart and lungs, causing collapse and death.

Although the model is simplistic, it does enable us to categorise our intakes.

But we have to be careful here. Some substances act like a food, but at high dosage could become a poison. A small amount of salt helps prevent us dehydrating, yet too much could be fatal.

However, there are substances that we are told are foods but should be classified as a poison.

- *Margarine and hydrogenated vegetable oil.* Although these have been around since the time of the Napoleonic wars, they became widely commercially available with the advent of modern methods of processing hydrogenated fats – now known as toxic trans-fats. These are known to cause coronary heart disease (Ascherio *et al.* 1999), diabetes and obesity, and to contribute to neurological disorders such as Alzheimer's (Morris *et al.* 2003) and many other diseases.

- *Aspartame.* This controversial artificial sweetener (scientific name *1-aspartyl 1-phenylalanine methyl ester*) was introduced commercially by NutraSweet, a subsidiary of Monsanto. Some researchers believe that eating artificial sweeteners stimulates desire for carbohydrates, thus negating efforts to lose weight.

  Aspartame is a known excitoxin (as is MSG – monosodium glutamate or E621) (Blaylock 1994). Excitotoxins are substances which can cause neurotoxicity and affect the functioning of the brain and nervous system. There is research suggesting that aspartame can affect brain chemistry, even altering people's behaviour (Wurtman 1983).

Furthermore, concerns have been raised about the increased use of this sweetener and a possible link to the greater prevalence of brain tumours (Olney *et al.* 1996). One study showed a relief in the symptoms of fibromyalgia after the exclusion of the excitotoxins MSG and aspartame from the diet (Smith *et al.* 2001).

- *High fructose corn syrup.* Not yet common in the UK, but present in some sports drinks and soft/fizzy drinks. It is creeping into biscuits and cereals and in the USA is commonplace in many foods, including most bread. I find it alarming that it is also being used more and more in baby formula milks. Some researchers suggest that high fructose corn syrup is responsible for the increase in overweight six-month-old babies. Children as young as three are now showing signs of heart disease (BBC 2010) and many observers are labelling this generation the 'children of the corn syrup'.

  Although it is a high glycaemia food (see page 45), high fructose corn syrup is not recognised by the body as a sugar. It disturbs insulin levels, leading many experts to believe that it has contributed to the increase in childhood diabetes. When you consume high fructose corn syrup it fools your brain into thinking that the body is starving, creating a condition called metabolic syndrome. The body does not process it like a sugar, but more like a fat. High fructose corn syrup:

  ○ makes you fat

  ○ increases cholesterol and causes a fatty liver

  ○ is toxic to the liver

  ○ causes gout

- ○ increases blood pressure

- ○ causes heart disease

- ○ causes diabetes.

  Your body processes any fructose like a poison; however, the effects are countered when taken with high fibre and vitamin C, so fruit is not a problem.

- *Fluoride.* The addition of fluoride to municipal water supplies to 'improve' dental health has long been a concern. There are many potential problems that can occur with an intake of fluoride, such as effects on bone density and bio-accumulation in the system. There is uncertainty as to what is a safe level of fluoride in water.

  - ○ Children exposed to high levels of fluoride in the water have been shown to have reduced IQ (Lu *et al.* 2000).

  - ○ Fluoride in drinking water is known to reduce fertility rates and have a disruptive effect on hormones in men (Freni 1994; Ortiz-Pérez *et al.* 2003).

  - ○ Fluoride exposure can decrease thyroid function and impair glucose tolerance (National Research Council 2006).

Other man-made hazards in our intake to watch out for include:

- additives and preservatives: although some are made from natural ingredients such as seaweed, others are from synthetic petrochemicals

- food wrapped in plastic

- food that is highly processed and cooked in a convenient way, such as microwaved

- fast foods, now dominating food culture in the Western world.

A SPOONFUL OF SUGAR MAKES THE MEDICINE GO DOWN

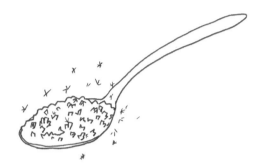

In 1830 the average person ate 5kg of sugar a year. In 2000 the average person ate 70kg of sugar a year (Servan-Schreiber 2009). That means an average of 36 teaspoons a day!

From World War II to the present day our intake of sugar has increased exponentially. Today, the primary source of calories in the US is sugar.

The intake of refined sugar is implicated in several disorders and conditions and is known to accelerate the ageing process. It has no nutritional value whatsoever; it is an empty calorie. And yet, given the choice between an artificial sweetener and sugar, I'd take sugar every time, such is the undesirability of aspartame. Some other major changes that have occurred since the end of World War II include:

- *Our food has a harmful ratio of nutrients.* The soil is depleted in minerals, farming is more intensive and more of our food is highly refined and processed. The balance of oils has changed from being high in omega 3 and low in omega 6 to low in omega 3 and high in omega 6. This ratio change in these essential fats contributes to inflammation and therefore disease.

- *Our food is exposed to more pesticides and man-made chemicals.* These include pesticides and fertilisers, while 'foods' such as hydrogenated fats, artificial sweeteners and high fructose corn syrup are substances that, as a species, we never ingested before.

- *Our diet has become high in refined sugar and the overall glycaemic index (see page 45) has been increased.*

- *We consume more animal products, such as meat and dairy.*

CHECKLIST FOR A HEALTHY APPROACH TO FOOD AND DRINK

Food:

- Eat organic food wherever possible.

- Reduce or cut out meat.

- If you have milk products, opt for grass-fed only and non-homogenised and non-pasteurised (raw). Raw dairy is more digestible.

- Avoid sugar and foods that are high on the glycaemic index (see page 45).

- Avoid processed food, instead opting for home-made meals and preparations.

Water:

- Avoid drinking water out of plastic.

- Filter your household water supply to reduce fluoride, insecticides and other contaminants.

- Use a charcoal or reverse osmosis filter.

- Place a water filter attachment to your shower, as many of the toxic compounds in mains water can be inhaled and absorbed through the skin.

Chapter 3

GUIDELINES FOR HEALTHY EATING

I recommend some basic guidelines to the diet we eat, in order to achieve optimum health.

There are two systems that I think are really helpful: the acid–alkaline balance and the glycaemic index.

Acid–alkaline balance

The acid–alkaline balance of our food affects the underlying biochemical balance within our body. pH is the scientific measure used to assess whether something is acid or alkaline. Pure water is neutral, with a pH of 7.0; substances with a pH of less than 7 are said to be acidic, while those with a pH of more than 7 are said to be alkaline.

Many holistic practitioners put great emphasis on the importance of eating a diet that is predominantly alkaline in nature, in order to treat and prevent ill health.

Acidity in the body produces a number of effects, including:

- inflammation

- reduced ability to detoxify.

If the pH range of a cell is too acidic, then cellular respiration is reduced. Basically, this means a decrease in the ability for nutrition to enter the cell to produce energy and toxins to be mobilised and expelled. When the pH balance goes awry these processes become compromised.

Too much acidity may contribute to conditions such as osteoporosis. When the body is acidic it causes demineralisation. The body uses the minerals stored in the body as a way to balance the pH. Medical anthropologist Dr Susan E. Brown, through cross-cultural research, found that those cultures who consumed the most amount of calcium in their diet had the highest incidence of osteoporosis-based fractures (Brown 2000). She attributes some of the high incidence of osteoporosis fractures in the Western world to our acidic diet, in which the body releases calcium from the bones and tissues into the blood in order to balance the pH. This was demonstrated in the Framingham Osteoporosis Study, which revealed that the intake of cola drinks is linked with lower bone density in older women (Tucker *et al.* 2006).

Glycaemic index

The concentration of glucose (sugar) in the blood is called glycaemia. A high concentration of sugar in the blood is called 'hyperglycaemia', and a low level 'hypoglycemia'. The body responds to the presence of glucose in the blood by excreting the hormone insulin, which facilitates its removal. This serves to maintain the correct levels of blood glucose.

However, different foods can have a lesser or greater effect on our blood glucose levels. The glycaemic index lets us know which foods these are.

WHY IS THIS IMPORTANT?

Every time we eat, the body regulates the sugar levels in the blood through insulin excretion. A diet that is rich in foods high on the glycaemic index (GI), such as refined carbohydrates and sugar, is constantly provoking the body to produce large amounts of insulin. What can occur over time is that the body becomes desensitised to the consistently high presence of insulin in the bloodstream. The body then gradually excretes more insulin to have the same effect. This is called insulin resistance.

This is a problem, as hyperinsulinism is associated with a myriad of health problems:

- cancer

- fatigue

- heart disease

- high blood pressure

- macular degeneration

- obesity.

To reduce the hyperinsulinism it is important to eat a diet which doesn't provoke a big insulin response. Essentially this means eating a diet which on the whole is low on the glycaemic index, that is, foods which are slow releasing carbohydrates. There is much literature written about how to eat according to the GI index, particularly by Michel Montignac (www.montignac.com). As you will notice in this simplified table, the more refined and processed, the higher on the GI it tends to be.

Table 3.1 Glycaemic index of foods

Low GI (55 or less)	Medium GI (56–69)	High GI (70 and above)
Fruit	Whole wheat products	Sugar
Most vegetables	Brown rice	White bread
Legumes/pulses	Sweet potato	White rice
Whole grains	Baked potatoes	Cornflakes
Nuts	Honey	Most breakfast cereals
Dairy	Banana	Glucose
Dark chocolate		Maltose
Rye bread		Beer
		Crisps
		Soft drinks

Foods that have an acidic effect on the body tend to be those from animals or foods which have been highly processed. It is wise to eat foods which are more alkaline such as vegetables and avoid those that create acidity such as refined carbohydrates and sugars.

Table 3.2 General guidelines for healthy eating

Foods to avoid or reduce – higher on the glycaemic index, pro-inflammatory, more acidic or higher in toxins	Foods that can be eaten more freely – tend to be lower on the glycaemic index, anti-inflammatory and more alkaline
Drinks	
Tap water Water stored in plastic Fruit juices made from concentrate or pasteurised smoothies Carbonated drinks, colas and squash	Filtered water, reverse osmosis, or carbon filter Clean well or spring water from the source Mineral water stored in glass bottles Herb teas, green tea, lemon water Fresh juices, vegetable and fruit
Vegetables	
Deep fried, boiled, and barbecued potatoes	Eaten raw, steamed, briefly stir fried: artichoke, beetroot, broccoli, cabbage, carrot, cauliflower, celery, cucumber, french beans, green beans, lettuce, parsnips, peas, peppers, pumpkin, rocket, spinach, sprouted beans and lentils, squash, sweet potato, watercress, yam, zuccini Sprouted beans and seeds
Grains and cereals	
White refined grains, such as wheat White pasta White rice White bread Refined and sugared cereals from corn, puffed rice, cornflakes	Whole grains Amaranth Brown rice Bulgar wheat Millet Oats Quinoa (alkaline) Rye bread

Fats and oils	
Trans-fats and hydrogenated oils (totally avoid)	Avocado
Corn oil	Ghee (from cow's butter)
Lard	Butter (grass-fed cattle)
Margarine	Flaxseed
Vegetable ghee	Extra virgin olive oil
Frying oils	Walnut oil
Corn oil, sunflower oil, peanut oil	Pumpkin oil
	Coconut oil

Dairy	
Homogenised, pasteurised cow's milk, semi-skimmed, skimmed and dairy products from corn-fed cattle	Raw, unpasteurised, unhomogenised whole organic milk and dairy products from grass-fed cows, goat's milk, ghee

Fruits	
Tinned fruits in syrup	Raspberries, blueberries, blackberries, blackcurrants, red currants

Sweeteners and sweet things	
Aspartame	Agave syrup, xylitol, stevia, black strap molasses, luo han guo (a very sweet tasting fruit that is low on the glycaemic index), raw honey
High fructose corn syrup (totally avoid)	
Saccharin	
White refined sugar	Dark chocolate with a minimum of 70 per cent cocoa solids
Honey which is cooked, maple syrup, malt syrup, sorbitol, saccharine, fructose, maltose, dextrose	Small amounts of unsulphured dried fruits such as raisins, dates, mangos and apples
Pastries and cakes	Fresh fruit can also be used as a sweetener, especially apples and pears

Protein	
All meat excepting fish	Lentils, beans, legumes and peas, tofu and fermented soya, tempeh, fish, eggs (organic/free range) (if needed while making a transition to a more plant-based diet)

Salt	
Table salt	Himalayan rock salt, sea salt, seaweed, miso, fermented soya sauce
Nuts and seeds	
Peanuts (high in mould), and nuts that have been roasted	Raw almonds, macadamia, Brazil nuts, apricot kernels, walnuts Flaxseeds/linseeds, pumpkin seeds, sunflower seeds
Herbs, spices and condiments	
Malt vinegar, table salt, MSG (monosodium glutamate), ketchup	Cider vinegar, turmeric, ginger, garlic, nigella seeds, black pepper, cayenne, tamari, nutritional yeast, fermented foods
Food source bacteria	
Antagonists to beneficial bacteria: tap water with chlorine and fluoride, antibiotics in medication and animal products, alcohol and some medical drugs such as the contraceptive pill	Beneficial micro-flora in the form of sauerkraut, kefir, kimchi, yoghurt, zoyers (pickled veg), idli (an Indian fermented black lentils and rice dish)

WE ARE GETTING FATTER

Interestingly, the percentage of calorie intake in the form of fat has decreased since the 1960s. One of the problems with the Western diet is *not* that we eating more fat, but that the intake of refined carbohydrates and sugars has increased. Refined carbohydrates and sugars increase the levels of insulin in the body, which in turn causes all kinds of effects such as:

- cardiovascular disease

- increased appetite, leading to overeating

- metabolic syndrome

- type II diabetes

- weight gain.

Fats

Unfortunately, over the years fats have gained a bad name. However, we need the good fats in our diet to keep healthy and fight disease. A low-fat diet is just as bad as a diet that is high in fat. The issue with fats is that there are different types, and the situation can become confusing. Fats are divided into:

- trans-fats
- saturated fats
- omega 3
- omega 6.

The Western diet has become increasingly high in the 'bad' fats. These contribute to inflammation in the body and disease.

Trans-fats

These are a complete no no. Created by the hydrogenation of oils, they are implicated in heart disease, cancer, diabetes, Alzheimer's… Basically, trans-fats are bad news. Some countries, including Denmark, have now banned the sale of hydrogenated oils. Hydrogenated oil is typically an ingredient in commercial pastries, bread, some margarines, cakes and biscuits.

Saturated fats

These are present in meat and dairy and in coconut oil. For years they have been implicated as the cause of heart and cardiovascular disease, although in many nutritional circles it is now believed that saturated fat is not the evil substance many believe it to be. Since the 1960s, governments around the world have emphatically stated that saturated fat is the cause of increased cholesterol, diabetes and heart disease.

Since then, there has been a disproportionate increase in the use of fried vegetable oil, refined carbohydrate and sugar in food. Although saturated fat intake has reduced in the developed world, heart disease and type II diabetes has steadily increased. It could be that saturated fat isn't the problem at all, but that people are eating food high in sugar, salt, refined carbohydrates and margarine.

Fat is important in the production of many hormones. For example, we make hormones from cholesterol and fat. Some saturated fat in our diet is important for our body to deal better with stress.

Omega 3 fatty acid

This essential fatty acid has massive implications for our level of health. It:

- helps the body resolve harmful fatty deposits
- helps to optimise the brain, cognitive function and mental health
- helps prevent cancer
- helps prevent autoimmune diseases
- helps keep eyes healthy
- helps keep the heart healthy
- helps keep the joints healthy
- helps to maintain the integrity of the cell membrane
- helps the body to create hormones.

Omega 6

This is also an essential fatty acid; however, most people's diet tends to be too dominant in this fat. If the diet is loaded in favour of omega 6 then there will be a tendency toward inflammation and a host of degenerative diseases. Its presence is high in fast foods, cakes, biscuits and fried foods.

The fatty acid balancing act

Although both omega 3 and omega 6 are needed by the body, the ratio of these oils has to be correct for us to be healthy. There is some debate as to what is the ideal ratio, but the diet should be at least equal in quantity of omega 3 and 6 fats. Most people need a ratio of 2:1 of omega 3 to omega 6, as there is usually inflammation present in the body. Unfortunately, the standard Western diet is completely distorted with a ratio of up to 50:1 of omega 6 to omega 3!

Omega 3 reduces inflammation in the body and has been shown to have anti-cancer properties and aids with detoxification. I would say that the majority of people are deficient in this important oil. Omega 3 has massive importance for health. It is present in:

- fish

- flaxseed oil

- fresh vegetables

- grass-fed organic dairy

- walnuts.

What about frying?

When oils are heated, the molecular structure of the oil changes. Each oil has an individual smoke point, at which the nutritional factors then begin to break down. Some oils are able to withstand a high temperature, whereas others are not. Oils that are heated up to beyond their smoke point become harmful to consume as they increase the formation of free radicals in the body.

Frying should only be done in oils which are semi-solid or hard at room temperature. This indicates that the oil will not break down as easily when heated to a high temperature.

Although I don't advocate a diet high in anything deep fried, frying should only be done with saturated fat:

- butter

- coconut oil

- ghee.

VEGETARIAN AND VEGAN DIETS

There are many cultures which are fundamentally vegetarian. India has a long tradition of vegetarianism, particularly amongst Jains, Buddhists and Hindus. There is also a tradition of veganism in some areas of China. 'Pure vegetarians' don't eat meat, fish or eggs. In these cultures there is normally a strong principle of ahimsa, or non-violence. A vegetarian or vegan diet certainly can be the right dietary choice for many people. Those following a strict spiritual path often find that committing to a vegetarian regime is instrumental to their development.

Following a vegetarian diet does, however, need careful consideration. It is important to make sure that you take vitamin B12 supplementation. Many people turn to the nutritional algae, spirulina. Although this is not a viable source of B12, it contains an analogue that mimics B12 in laboratory tests (see the section on vitamin B12 on page 63). B12 is also a common deficiency for meat eaters.

If you are vegetarian it is important to not over-consume carbohydrates in the form of grains or refined sugar. I have experienced that vegetarians who are not eating enough protein for their body type will instead crave sugar. Indian cuisine has a lot to offer in the form of Ayurvedic cooking, which will help you to eat enough absorbable vegetable protein, and has developed techniques which support the body in being vegetarian. For example, lentils properly cooked with spices and herbs can be well digested, but if they are not then they can cause bloating, wind and discomfort.

If you can tolerate dairy, then that can be a healthy addition to the diet, especially in the form of ghee or clarified cow butter. However, dairy should be organic, non-homogenised, grass-fed and raw. Goat milk is often more easily digested, as is dairy from sheep.

Soya

Turning to soya as a protein might not be a great idea either. Soya has oestrogenic qualities and can affect thyroid function. Tofu, which is made from soya, is normally fine for most people to eat once or twice a week, but I wouldn't advocate daily intake of soya, especially for males. You often find vegetarian meals laden with soya, so that soya is being consumed multiple times a day. For most, a little (non-GM) soya is fine, but don't overdo it, and I think it should be avoided in boys. In China, soya has traditionally been eaten in its fermented form, which predigests it and makes it more digestible and resolves many of the problematic nutritional factors.

Vegetarians and sugar

Long term, I don't think it is possible to be a healthy vegetarian while still consuming refined sugar. I have seen sugar intake being much more detrimental to vegetarians than even to meat eaters. In the Chinese Taoist tradition it is stated that monks needing to be vegetarian also need to take tonic herbs to keep healthy. Many of these tonic herbs are a source of B12, such as dong quai (*Angelica sinensis*). In Ayurvedic medicine, daily tonic herbs support healthy digestive enzyme production and specifically healthy stomach acid levels. It is vital for vegetarians and vegans that stomach acid levels are kept at the right pH, so that proteins can be properly broken down and digested (see page 82).

Raw food

The principle of raw food is that by eating produce that has not been cooked or processed it will speed up your body's ability to repair and heal itself. Many will eat a diet of raw sprouted beans, salad, raw vegetables, vegetable smoothies, and some fruit. Other additions may be herbal powders in the smoothies such as spirulina, maca (*Lepidium meyenii*) and chlorella. Many in the living food movement consider it to have been started by Ann Wigmore (1909–1994), who nursed thousands of people back to health using wheatgrass juice and living foods. A colleague of mine, Elaine Bruce, routinely teaches people the art of preparing living food and how to incorporate it into your life.

Some people do well on a diet of living food as it is excellent for detoxification, or for certain degenerative conditions. However, I normally recommend it for only short periods of time. I think it is certainly sustainable in hot and dry countries, but in a cold, wet climate most people need to find a healthy percentage of cooked food in their diet.

NECESSARY NUTRIENTS

At school we are taught about the main food groups: carbohydrates, protein, sugars and fats. We may have been told that we need to eat a balanced diet in order for our body to function properly, and learnt about the role of calories and salt. Other nutrients may have been mentioned, along with how a lack of them in our diet can cause certain diseases: vitamin C and scurvy; iron and anaemia; calcium and osteoporosis; vitamin D and rickets. But usually it is at that point our nutritional education ends.

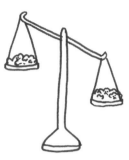

There is huge emphasis on macronutrients, the nuts and bolts of our diet: carbohydrates, iron, calcium, protein. There is very little emphasis on trace elements or micronutrients. However, researching the role these micronutrients play shows that not only are they fundamental for the functioning of our body, but that without them we cannot treat or prevent disease.

I test my patients for trace elements and the levels of vitamins and essential fatty acids. Again and again I find a familiar pattern, that of certain mineral and vitamin deficiencies.

Recommended daily allowance

The UK's recommended daily allowance (RDA) is the basic nutritional requirement the body needs to function. However, those of us who work in the field of nutrition know that for many, the basic nutritional intake is often not enough to prevent illness and manage pre-existing conditions. Our body is being put under increasingly bigger demands in the form of pollution, stress, or ongoing infections and imbalances. To tackle these stressors we experience, it is understandable that we may need more than the RDA to be in healthy equilibrium.

More minerals

It is no wonder, considering the depleted condition of the soil that our food is grown from, that mineral deficiency is at epidemic proportions.

ZINC

The blood tests of my patients reveal that people are almost universally short of zinc. Why is this such a big deal? Zinc is necessary for the production of stomach acid, which in turn breaks down protein into amino acids for absorption. From this we make all kinds of neurotransmitters: serotonin, melatonin, dopamine and many others. If we don't have enough zinc a whole complex chain of events cannot occur properly and we don't produce enough brain chemicals. Without sufficient quantities of zinc in our body we cannot absorb and utilise essential fatty acids even if we are consuming them.

The result can be feeling depressed, anxious, unable to concentrate and left vulnerable to developing all kinds of psychiatric symptoms. We can develop problems with our hormones and nervous system and furthermore are predisposed to a whole host of diseases and immune insufficiency.

Zinc is available in:

- alfalfa sprouts
- nettles
- seeds, especially pumpkin and sunflower.

If you have had your levels tested and they are low, and you want to take a supplement, it is worth taking it in liquid form to ensure good absorption.

SELENIUM

Selenium is a vital mineral which has cancer-protective effects. It is also important in the production of the thyroid hormone, thyroxin. It plays an important role in protecting against autoimmune disease, which is a common cause of a malfunctioning thyroid gland. It helps to protect us from heavy metals and is important in detoxification. The most reliable source of selenium is Brazil nuts.

MAGNESIUM

Magnesium deficiency is so common that it warrants a bit more of an explanation. At any one time the body contains about 25g of magnesium, about 12g of which is contained in the bones, with the rest in the nerves, organs and blood. It is an essential mineral, and has many functions:

- It enables healthy cell replication and repair.

- It is essential in hormonal production.

- It activates B vitamins.

- It is necessary for bone health.

- It is involved in at least 300 enzyme processes.

- It helps with transmission of nerve impulses.

- It relaxes muscles.

- It has a role in the production of insulin.

- It is needed for production of ATP (adrenosine triphosphate), which is responsible for cellular energy.

A chronic deficiency of magnesium is common, where the body does not have adequate stores in the cells. More and more research is revealing that having enough magnesium reserves in your body is essential not only for preventing and managing certain diseases but also for having enough physical energy.

Magnesium is absolutely essential for the human body to function. Intensive farming methods and the consumption of refined foods is resulting in a large-scale deficiency, insidiously degrading many people's health.

Even though the RDA of vitamins and minerals is often far too low for most people, studies have shown that many people don't even meet the RDA requirement for magnesium. An example is a study conducted on patients in intensive care units which revealed that two-thirds were deficient in the mineral (Weisinger and Bellorin-Font 1998).

Magnesium deficiency is associated with heart disease, arthritis, chronic fatigue and depression and many other disorders. Magnesium plays a crucial role in:

- dilating the bronchioles (useful in childhood asthma)

- preventing hardening of the arteries

- maintaining healthy cholesterol levels

- regulating the rhythm of the heart

- promoting healthy detoxification of cells

- producing serotonin, a neurotransmitter that gives us a sense of wellbeing

- flushing toxins such as heavy metals from cells.

Magnesium researcher Paul Mason (1994) states: 'Magnesium deficiency appears to have caused 8 million sudden coronary deaths in America during the period 1940–1994.' He is campaigning for all bottled drinks to be supplemented with magnesium.

The symptoms of magnesium deficiency include:

- ADHD

- anxiety

- arthritis

- asthma
- calcification of tissues
- cold extremities
- constipation
- chronic fatigue
- cramps
- depression
- headaches
- high blood pressure
- insomnia
- kidney stones
- migraines
- muscle cramps, tics, twitches, tremors
- PMS.

With any of these symptoms and conditions, magnesium levels should be checked to see if it has a role to play.

Magnesium deficiency affects people on all kinds of diets; however, the more refined the diet the more deficient one tends to be.

Research by Cox *et al.* (1991) has shown that people with chronic fatigue have low levels of red blood cell magnesium. In the same study, when levels were appropriately restored, many of those with fatigue felt an increase in energy as well as being more able to deal with their emotions.

A study in China by Slutsky *et al.* 2010 showed that high levels of magnesium supplementation improve cognitive brain function and the brain's ability to adapt and cope with stress.

Reasons for magnesium deficiency include:

- *Low dietary magnesium.* Intake is simply not enough. This is likely, especially as the soil in so many areas is depleted in minerals.

- *Insufficient stomach acid.* Many people, especially those with chronic disease, do not have a strong enough concentration of acid, resulting in poor protein metabolism as well as mineral deficiencies such as iron. Stomach acid concentration can decrease as we get older, decreasing the absorption of minerals.

- *Sweating and exercise.* Athletes and those doing intense exercise have a greater need for magnesium. Many believe it is magnesium deficiency that causes 'sudden death syndrome'.

- *Stress.* At times of acute stress the need for magnesium is greater.

- *Diuretics.* These leach magnesium from the body. In addition to medication, diuretics also include tea and coffee.

Alcoholics and diabetics all have a greater need for magnesium. Magnesium can be obtained from:

- *Seaweeds.* High in magnesium.

- *Chocolate.* High in magnesium. In my experience people who crave chocolate are almost always magnesium deficient.

- *Nuts and seeds.* Cashews, almonds, pumpkin and sesame seeds.

- *Chlorophyll.* At the centre of the chlorophyll molecule is a magnesium atom. Chlorophyll gives plants their green colour, so the greener the better. Ideal sources are wheatgrass, kale and spinach as well as 'superfoods' like spirulina and chlorella.

THE DYNAMIC DUO

So much is talked about calcium and it is frequently the main concern when people change their diet, especially if they are avoiding dairy. However, the question is never, 'Will I get enough magnesium?'

There is a careful balance between calcium and magnesium in the body. These minerals compete for absorption. It is considered that our calcium/magnesium need is a ratio of 2:1. Cow dairy has a ratio of 12:1, which is why some practitioners conclude that a high consumption of dairy products could result in magnesium deficiency.

Where calcium causes muscles and nerves to contract, magnesium relaxes. Magnesium allows calcium to be absorbed into the bones rather than it building up in the soft tissues of the body. Common results of a high calcium and low magnesium intake in the diet are kidney stones, calcium spurs and hardening of the arteries, yet the bones may still be weak. So in some cases of osteoporosis, using calcium as a supplement will not help, as it could further upset the mineral balance of the body.

We need the correct amount of magnesium in order for the heart to function properly. Calcium supplementation without the intake of magnesium will upset the balance. This would explain why, when a group of older women who took calcium supplements were studied, it was discovered that they were at greater risk of heart attacks (Bolland *et al.* 2011; Cox, Campbell and Dowson 1991; Slutsky *et al.* 2010).

Magnesium supplementation

Overall, magnesium is a safe supplement. It comes in a variety of forms, the most common being magnesium oxide, although I have found magnesium citrate to be a very absorbable form. In the European Union, the RDA of magnesium is 375mg a day. If a healthy person overdoses on magnesium it will result in diarrhoea.

However, depending on individual biochemical factors, an individual might need more than the RDA. Testing is the most reliable way to determine what you need.

Taking homeopathic remedies can help to increase the absorption of certain minerals. The homeopathic tissue salt 'Mag Phos' can be taken to increase the absorption of the mineral and is especially good for when someone is getting cramps and spasms.

Magnesium supplementation is not recommended for people with kidney disease.

Magnesium baths

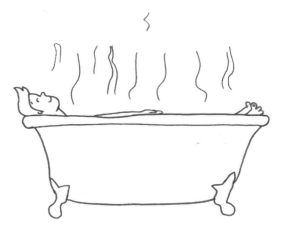

An easy and very effective way to replenish your levels of magnesium is by soaking in an Epsom salts (magnesium sulphate) bath. In this way magnesium can be absorbed into the body through the skin.

Although Epsom salts baths have been used medicinally for hundreds of years, only recently has a full study of its properties been conducted. Researchers at Birmingham University, England, measured the increase of magnesium in blood plasma after soaking in a bath of Epsom salts. They found that it is best absorbed when the solution is approximately 1 per cent Epsom salts to water. This equates to 500–600 grams of salts for the average domestic bath, a concentration that feels slightly soapy. There were no perceived side-effects in the study and two of the volunteers taking part reported that their rheumatic pains disappeared.

The researchers concluded that, 'Bathing in Epsom salts is a safe and easy way to increase magnesium levels in the body' (Waring 2004).

Tips to improve magnesium levels

- Have an Epsom salts bath once a week.

- Eat chlorophyll-rich food in the form of wheatgrass, spirulina, chlorella and leafy green vegetables.

- If you are taking a calcium supplement make sure you also take magnesium.

- Add black pepper to your meals. Studies have shown that it can massively increase the absorption of what it is eaten with.

- Make sure you are eating enough good fats and a diet high in antioxidants. Healthy cell membranes keep magnesium within the cells.

Testing for magnesium

The different ways of testing magnesium levels include testing urine, sweat and blood. The blood serum test is the most routine method of testing, and measures how much magnesium there is in the blood. It is important to monitor this, as it is vital that the body keeps magnesium levels in the blood finely balanced and within a very narrow range in order for the body to function and for the heart to continue functioning. Magnesium from within the cells' reserves and also the bones will be drawn upon to keep the levels in the blood constant.

For our purposes the red cell magnesium test is the most useful for analysing chronic deficiency as it measures the level of magnesium in the cells, which is indicative of your reserves. Frequently the red cell magnesium test will determine that red cell levels are deficient, even though the blood serum test has indicated that serum levels are within the normal range.

Case history: Cluster headaches

Adam (52) came to the clinic because he was suffering from cluster headaches. They were so severe that when he had an attack he would need to spend at least five days in bed. Cluster headaches are known for being one of the most painful disorders imaginable. For him they began when he was about 13 and he would have an episode every two to three months. Over the years he tried many different diets and treatments – some helped a little bit, but nothing gave him a permanent solution. After testing his magnesium levels I discovered that although his serum levels were normal his intracellular levels (i.e. within the cells) were very low. He embarked on supplementation of magnesium in various forms. Remarkably, after six months he hadn't had an attack, and 18 months later he still hasn't had a cluster headache.

Vitamin B12

Another important nutritional factor is B12. It is often not taken seriously enough by either orthodox or alternative health professionals. I will explain why it is so vital that you get enough of this vitamin, why I believe it is best to get tested regularly and why, if you are deficient, it is essential you take steps, as untreated B12 deficiency can cause irreparable damage.

WHAT IS B12?

Vitamin B12, also called cobalamin, is needed to create red blood cells, to enable folic acid absorption and utilisation, and for a healthy nervous system and brain. It also acts as a co-enzyme, enabling healthy DNA replication to take place, as well as the metabolism of amino acids and fats. It is essential for the maintenance of the myelin sheath, which is the layer that surrounds the nerves. The body can store B12 for a period of two to five years, and 80 per cent of storage is in the liver. Its presence in the body is vital for the breakdown of homocysteine, therefore essential for healthy detoxification.

There are a number of sources of B12. It is present in meat, fish and dairy products; it is also present in some yeasts and in bacterially rich environments such as soil.

Vegetarians and vegans are at a greater risk of B12 deficiency than the rest of the population, as B12 is almost exclusively obtainable from animal products. Grains, vegetables, fruits, pulses, nuts and seeds do not contain any B12.

In many parts of Asia vegetarianism has been practised successfully for thousands of years. People relied on fermented foods, which were created in an environment where B12-rich bacteria dominated. These included foods such as tempeh, miso and soy sauce. Because of strict hygiene standards, fermented foods commercially produced in the West have virtually no naturally occurring B12. Many manufacturers have realized this and more recently have started supplementing their products.

IT'S NOT HOW MUCH YOU EAT – IT'S HOW MUCH YOU ABSORB

Even if you are consuming enough B12, deficiencies can occur if the body is not absorbing enough of it. In order for B12 to be absorbed through the small intestine, it needs to be combined with 'intrinsic factor', a substance produced in the stomach. Some people are unable to create intrinsic factor and they become B12 deficient. This leads to a condition called pernicious anaemia.

Reasons for impaired B12 absorption are:

- a lack of intrinsic factor, which is believed to be caused by a hereditary autoimmune disorder

- deterioration of the stomach lining, including ulcers (more common in the over-50s)

- age – as we get older our ability to absorb B12 usually decreases

- irritable bowel syndrome, inflammatory bowel diseases or unidentified coeliac disease

- bacterial infections in the gut

- certain drugs can interfere with absorption, such as antacids, proton pump inhibitors and the diabetic drug metformin

- mercury and anaesthetics can interfere with absorption, and levels can be low because of parasitic infestation such as tapeworm

- gastric operations, such as removal of sections of the gut.

Symptoms of pernicious anaemia are the same as those of iron-deficient anaemia and include fatigue, pale skin and breathlessness. A blood test in this instance would usually reveal enlarged red blood cells. If someone has the classic signs and symptoms of pernicious anaemia, effective treatment can prevent them from a whole collection of serious and debilitating health problems. Pernicious anaemia is usually easily detected and treated either through B12 injections and/or high doses of oral supplementation.

There is a big 'but' here. A third of people with B12 deficiency never develop the usual blood abnormalities of large red blood cells or anaemia. A full blood count from your doctor doesn't include testing for B12 levels in the blood. Usually B12 is only tested when the red blood cells are unusually large, and someone can have low B12 levels without this sign being present. Symptoms are often misdiagnosed, leading to potentially devastating consequences. If someone's levels are low then they have probably been depleting their reserves for a number of years.

EFFECTS OF B12 DEFICIENCY

B12 deficiency can sometimes exhibit itself with a dull pale or yellow tint to the skin. It can begin with subtle symptoms like occasional tiredness and apathy and can gradually develop into irreversible psychiatric and nervous system degeneration, dementia and eventual death. However, just because someone has a number of these symptoms doesn't necessarily mean they are caused by a lack of B12. It is important to also investigate other possible causes. Equally, B12 deficiency can mimic the symptoms of multiple sclerosis and other neurological disorders. Symptoms that may be observed are listed below.

Mental/psychological:

- apathy
- confusion
- delayed development in children
- dementia
- depression (especially post-natal)
- deterioration of mental health, mood swings, paranoia and other personality changes

- memory loss
- violent and irrational behaviour.

Neurological:

- abnormal neurological sensations, numbness, tingling and weakness
- balance problems
- incontinence
- pain
- paralysis
- restless legs
- tinnitus
- tremors
- vision loss.

Other symptoms:

- chronic fatigue
- disturbed appetite
- gastro-intestinal issues, constipation and diarrhoea
- insomnia
- sore tongue
- susceptibility to viral and bacterial infections
- tiredness
- vitiligo.

Low levels of B12 increase the levels of homocysteine in the blood. High levels of homocysteine have been associated with an increased risk of:

- Alzheimer's disease

- cardiovascular disease and strokes

- cancer

- osteoporosis.

Case history: B12 deficiency

Janet came to see me complaining of fatigue, depression, menstrual irregularity, poor memory and phases of hair loss. She had been vegetarian for 20 years, but had recently been craving meat. Tests by her doctor had shown her full blood count to be normal, with no anaemia detected. She was referred to a psychiatrist. When I first saw Janet, she had a number of other health issues, including a fungal dysbiosis in her gut. However, I suspected that she was low in B12. She had a blood test with her GP and it came back within normal limits, although at 206ng/l it was at the lower end of the normal spectrum. As well as tackling her digestive issues, I suggested a large amount of B12 taken in liquid sublingually every day, and a re-test in three months.

Fortunately her next blood test showed an increase to 350ng/l. She reported that her energy had increased dramatically, hair loss had stopped and she was feeling less depressed. However, because she had been depleted for possibly many years, I suggested continuing with the high levels of supplementation for another six months, followed by another blood test. It might be that she will need high-dose supplementation for 18 months or more to replenish her reserves. She continues to improve.

SOURCES OF B12

Because B12 is not found in plant foods, it is vital to supplement the diet daily. I have come across many people who have been vegetarian for 10 or 20 years and then start to crave meat, reporting that they feel better after they go back to eating animal products. I find that this is almost always caused by B12 deficiency and that once levels are restored they can continue to follow a vegetarian diet and be healthy again.

It is a common misconception that spirulina, chlorella and blue-green algae, despite having important nutritional components, are a good source of B12. These superfoods contain B12 analogues which when tested mimic true B12; however, when they are taken to treat B12 deficiency they are not effective. Nutritional yeast, however, does contain true B12 and can be useful as a non-animal source.

Soil is rich in bacteria and B12; there is no doubt that our modern day obsession with cleanliness has contributed to the epidemic of B12 deficiency and other health problems.

To make sure intake is sufficient, my recommendation is to take a B12 supplement every day. The RDA of B12 is about 1.5 micrograms a day. I suggest that this is rarely enough, and as discussed, it is all about absorption. With my patients I usually recommend a minimum daily dose of 50 micrograms, in the form of tablets or in liquid form. However, some people need as much as 2000 micrograms a day. Getting a blood test will be a good indicator, giving you valuable information as to the levels you personally need.

There is also a B12 skin patch which is reported to deliver 1000 micrograms into the bloodstream. I also use these with patients and have found them to be useful. High-dose injections of B12 (1000 to 2000 micrograms daily) are important for patients with pernicious anaemia or those who have had gastric surgery, although other people may need injections, especially if deficiency is severe and has been present for a long time. This is the quickest way to restore levels in the body, and is sometimes clinically necessary. In extreme cases it may be necessary to have an injection every day for a month, gradually tapering down to once a week and then once a month before normal levels are achieved.

B12 is also known for its energising effects. Many athletes and music artists use them to prevent getting adrenal burnout. Some famous chess champions are known to take them on tournament days to improve their concentration. There is no known toxicity dose of B12 (Higdon 2003) and excess levels are easily broken down and excreted from the body. There is a rare genetic condition called Leber's optic neuropathy where B12 in the form of cyanocobalamin is contraindicated; however, in this circumstance a form called hydroxycobalamin is usually given.

GETTING TESTED

Some people think that as long as they're taking a B12 supplement every day they are fine and protected. However, this isn't always true. I suggest that everyone, especially vegetarians, vegans and those on a living food diet, have an annual B12 blood test. In the UK this is usually as straightforward as requesting this test from your doctor or practice nurse, explaining that you are vegetarian.

Remember that a full blood count is not sufficient, as many mistakenly believe that B12 deficiency only shows up as large and misshapen red blood cells. The UK guidelines for appropriate blood levels are 200 nanograms per litre to 1000ng/l. Some researchers have discovered that symptoms and nervous system damage can begin to develop when levels are below 300ng/l and symptoms do not always disappear until levels are in excess of 600ng/l.

A small percentage of people need a higher than average level of B12 to function normally. This can mean that although blood tests reveal adequate levels, they in fact need much more and can benefit from extra supplementation. I have seen a number of patients who have recovered from chronic fatigue through taking large amounts of B12 (100mg daily), even though blood levels were well within the normal range.

There is a further test, which measures urinary MMA, or methylmalonic acid, levels. This test measures B12 activity at the tissue/cellular level, since MMA levels are directly related to a B12-dependent metabolic pathway. If there is elevated MMA, then there is B12 deficiency even if blood plasma levels are normal.

If in any doubt, I suggest that you consult a health professional who is fully aware of all the issues involved with B12 deficiency. There are many thousands of people eating a vegetarian or even a meat-based diet who are unaware that they may have a health time bomb ticking away inside them. Some think they are just suffering from the effects of old age, or feeling unusually tired and lethargic. Others may already have neurological symptoms or have developed mental health disorders.

THE WONDERS OF FERMENTED FOODS

There is a worldwide tradition of eating foods which have gone through a fermenting process. Creating fermented foods is an ancient practice, with evidence that they were consumed in Babylon some 7000 years ago. There is good reason why they have featured as an important part of almost all traditional diets around the world.

Fermented beverages are common in most cultures in the form of alcohol. This is usually made with something sweet such as fruit juice made from grapes, apples, berries, bananas, and so on. Fermentation then takes place with the presence of yeast, creating a by-product of alcohol and carbon dioxide.

For medicinal benefit we are interested in foods that have been fermented. These foods go through transformation with the presence of bacteria, and have significant health benefits. Fermented foods are a treasure trove of beneficial bacteria or micro-flora. Although most of these support digestive functions, others actively support immunity.

Many of the fermented foods are high in vitamin C and have been a valuable source of nutrients. In the age before refrigeration, fermentation was a way of preserving vegetables, especially in the winter months.

The micro-flora in bacteria-fermented foods support digestive function and have other protective effects such as reducing the incidence of diarrhoea, which is incredibly important in certain environments.

Fermented foods also increase the absorption of minerals in food. Phytic acid, present in grains and especially in soya, prevents the absorption of many nutrients. However, fermentation breaks down the phytic acid present in soya and other grains, making them much more digestible and increasing their nutrient benefit.

Our bacteria-obsessed society is making us less prone to some infections but ultimately we are developing more chronic conditions such as asthma and allergies. Utilising this ancient food and medicine is relatively easy.

Sauerkraut

In Eastern Europe, and especially Germany, there is a long history of consuming fermented cabbage. Sour cabbage or sauerkraut was taken by Captain James Cook on his sea voyages as it prevented scurvy. The Germans were commonly known as 'Krauts' because they used the fermented dish to prevent vitamin C deficiency, just as the British were called 'Limeys' as they ate limes for the same reason. The process that the cabbage goes through is called lacto-fermentation.

There are three fermentation stages that occur in sauerkraut production:

Cabbage – salt – water

⇓

Coliform bacteria initiate the fermentation
process and produce acid.

⇓

The acid gives rise to *Leuconostoc* bacteria.

⇓

Changes in pH enable the proliferation of *Lactobacillus* bacteria.

The end result is the presence of many diverse bacteria, including:

- *Leuconostoc mesenteroides*
- *Lactobacillus plantarum*
- *Pediococcus pentosaceus*
- *Lactobacillus brevis*
- *Leuconostoc citreum*
- *Leuconostoc argentinum*
- *Leuconostoc fallax*
- *Lactobacillus paraplantarum*
- *Lactobacillus coryniformis*
- *Weissella sp.*

(Plengvidhya *et al.* 2007)

How to make sauerkraut

Fermentation is ideally carried out in heavy ceramic or glass jars. It is easier to make a larger amount than a small amount. You will need:

a wide-mouthed glass or stone/ceramic jar

2–3 tbsp sea salt or rock salt (preferably Himalayan rock salt)

2 large cabbages

a cloth cover

1. Take off the outer leaves of the cabbage and finely grate the cabbage into a large bowl.

2. As you grate, mix the salt into the finely grated leaves.

3. Start putting the mixture into the jar. Put in a few tablespoons at a time so you can pack it down firmly into the jar with a wooden spatula. The salt draws the water out of the cabbage through the process of osmosis, enabling fermentation to happen.

4. The jar needs to be covered in order for the cabbage to stay submerged in the cabbage juice and salt solution. You should find something that will fit snugly in the jar, such as a saucer or another jar. A weight (such as a jam jar of water) should be put on top to keep the cabbage solution submerged.

5. After a few hours check that the juice is covering the leaves, and make sure that the weight is heavy enough.

6. Cover the whole set-up with a large cloth to keep dust out.

7. Store it somewhere cool, not in the refrigerator, but outside the back door, in the cellar or in a cupboard.

8. Next day, lift the lid and again make sure there is enough juice covering the cabbage. If there isn't, then the sauerkraut won't ferment but could rot. Add water as necessary.

9. Every few days, check the level of salt solution to make sure the mixture is covered.

10. The taste will get stronger the longer it ferments; also the warmer the environment it is stored in the quicker the fermentation. If you leave it on a kitchen worktop, therefore, the process will be quicker.

11. After two weeks the fermentation will usually be complete, and you will end up with a tangy cabbage mixture. Usually there will be some mould on top, so simply skim it off.

There are many variations and additions that can be made to the recipe, such as adding herbs, juniper berries, bay leaves, garlic and onions.

The completed sauerkraut can be stored in the fridge and will keep for at least three to four months. Take a tablespoon a day.

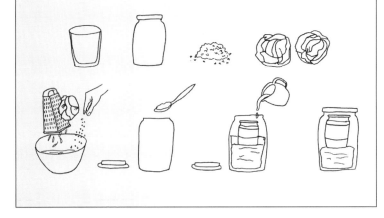

Case history: Sauerkraut

I noticed an interesting phenomenon in my clinic as I was treating a number of patients who had previously lived in Eastern Europe in countries such as Poland and the Ukraine and had settled in the UK in the last few years. Although the climate was much colder in the winter in their previous country, many had reported that after a year or two living in the UK they would begin to get much more frequent colds or more severe infections, especially in the winter months. They couldn't understand why this was. However, the answer came down to bacteria. At home, usually an older family member such as a grandmother would regularly make a fermented food such as sauerkraut. This would be eaten almost every day with the main meal. Upon living in the UK, they would still eat sauerkraut but it would be bought from a shop. One of the issues with commercially available sauerkraut is that it is most likely to be pasteurised and therefore lacking in all of the important micro-flora.

I would encourage these patients to make their own or get regular shipments from their grandmother. I then observed that infection rates dramatically reduced and their general immunity improved.

The benefits of good bacteria, such as those that are produced during the fermentation process, are only just being understood, but it is known to be important for:

- digestive health
- immunity
- improved mineral absorption
- reduction in inflammatory processes

- preventing infections such as from *Clostridium difficile*, *Salmonella*, *E. coli*

- lowering high blood pressure.

Case history: Fungal toenails

'I have suffered with fungal toe nails for at least ten years and although I tried all kinds of remedies, nothing worked, so I gave up trying anything else. I recently got into taking sauerkraut as I heard it was good for healthy digestion. I noticed that after three months of taking it my fungal nails completely cleared up! It must be the good bacteria.'

Chapter 4

THE DIGESTIVE SYSTEM
Nutrition In, Waste Out

On the wheel of health, the first spoke is related to nourishment and the second spoke is related to detoxification. Of course they are not entirely separate functions. I shall discuss both together here, as the process of breaking down foods into nourishment and the filtering away of waste are so interdependent and mutually supportive. Although the digestive system is comprised of a number of complicated processes, for our purpose we can see it as the absorption of nutrients and the elimination of waste. Let us travel through this remarkable system.

Digestion begins usually with the smell and anticipation of food. Saliva and digestive juices are stimulated and the body prepares for food.

As we chew we break food down into a semi-liquefied state. The saliva contains an enzyme called amylase, which starts to break down the carbohydrates ready for the sugars to be absorbed.

Once swallowed, it takes a few seconds for the food to be delivered into the stomach by a tube known as the oesophagus, or gullet. At the bottom of this tube is a valve, or sphincter, which prevents food and acid in the stomach entering the oesophagus.

The stomach then transforms the semi-liquid food into a substance called chyme. Food is broken down by hydrochloric acid, produced by the parietal cells in the stomach, which plays a vital role in the digestion of protein and also kills any unwanted bacteria or pathogens that might be present in the food. It is at this point that some absorption occurs directly from the stomach into the bloodstream, primarily liquids such as water and alcohol. The parietal cells also produce 'intrinsic factor', which enables us to absorb vitamin B12 later on in the gut. Pepsin, manufactured by the stomach, contributes to the breaking down of protein.

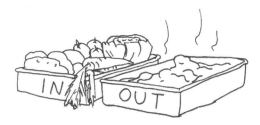

A thick layer of protective mucous prevents the stomach from digesting itself.

After about two hours, the chyme moves into the duodenum, which is the first section of the small intestine and is about two feet long. The pancreas secretes digestive enzymes such as amalyse, protease and lipase into the small intestine to promote further digestion of proteins, fats and carbohydrates, ready for absorption into the bloodstream. The pancreas also produces a substance similar to bicarbonate of soda which neutralises much of the acidity in the chyme so as to protect the small intestine.

Simultaneously, the liver and gallbladder excrete bile into the small intestine. Bile is an alkaline substance that changes fats into a water-soluble substance so they can be absorbed.

The chyme, which now has enzymes from the pancreas and bile and salts from the liver and gallbladder added, is ready for the next phase – absorption through the small intestine into the bloodstream.

The small intestine is some 20 feet long and is covered with tiny microvilli, which facilitate the absorption of nutrients. There is a part of the lining of the gut called the tight junctions, which serves to prevent the absorption of the wrong kinds of proteins and toxic by-products of digestion.

Different nutrients are absorbed in different sections of the small intestine. The small intestine contains millions of beneficial bacteria which increase the absorption of nutrients and maintain the correct balance between good and bad bacteria. Bad bacteria, such as *Salmonella*, which have not been killed by the stomach acids are rendered inert by the good bacteria.

In the resulting mixture that has now passed through the small intestine is a combination of fibre, water, bacteria and some unabsorbed nutrients. It then transits to the ileocaecal valve. This keeps the waste matter in the large intestine from passing back into the small intestine.

Our food now enters the colon, or large intestine. This is usually about four feet long. The large intestine will reabsorb three-quarters of the water remaining in the chyme to form faeces. Faeces are composed of approximately 30 per cent bacteria, with the rest made up of fibre, food particles and water. It can take up to 18 hours to pass through the large intestine.

At the end of the large intestine is the rectum, which contains two rings of muscles, or sphincters. The inner sphincter opens when a sufficient quantity of faeces has gathered to have a bowel movement. This is what gives us the feeling of wanting to evacuate our bowels. We then allow the outer sphincter, or the anus, to open, allowing the faeces to exit our body. The whole process from when the food is first consumed until the waste leaves the body ordinarily takes between 18 and 24 hours.

WHAT CAN GO WRONG

With our bodies comprised of such complex organs, it seems a miracle to me that, for the most part, they can carry out processes repeatedly without serious problems.

FOOD — A JOURNEY SUMMARISED

In the mouth
Food is broken down, assisted by the enzyme amylase in saliva.

⇓

In the stomach
Proteins are broken down with hydrochloric acid and pepsin, creating chyme.

⇓

At the small intestine
The pancreas excretes the enzymes amalyse, protease and lipase to digest protein and carbohydrates. The gallbladder and liver excrete bile for the digestion of fats. Absorption of nutrients takes place through the microvilli, while the absorption of harmful incompletely digested particles and microbes is prevented.

⇓

At the large intestine
Water is absorbed from the chyme leaving the end product, faeces.

⇓

At the rectum and anus
Faeces leave the body.

Most problems in the gut usually make themselves known through mild symptoms before serious discomfort occurs. Some symptoms are easily traced to the digestive system because they are felt during its function or around the direct area of the organs in question.

A healthy digestive system is the foundation of not only good digestive function but also the health of your whole body. In my clinic the most common complaints I come across are symptoms such as irritable bowel syndrome, inflammatory bowel disease and constipation. However, when the digestive function is under par it can also give rise to many other symptoms and disorders which may seem unrelated.

In many ways digestion begins when we see, smell and anticipate food. Our digestive juices start flowing and our body prepares for a meal. It is well known that the more appetising our food looks and smells, the increased capacity we have to digest it.

The action of chewing is one of the most important aspects of digestion. As mentioned, enzymes in saliva begin to break down starches as the digestive process begins. Usually, food stays in the stomach for about two hours while it is being broken down.

In the stomach there is a concentration of hydrochloric acid, which is produced by the parietal cells of the stomach lining. The pH of this acid should be between 1.8 and 2.6. This is incredibly acidic; if you got it directly on your skin it would burn. If it weren't for the presence of a layer of mucous coating the stomach, the acid would attack and start to digest the stomach wall.

The hydrochloric acid (HCl) serves a number of functions. This bath of acid enables the proteins to be broken down into the individual amino acids so that they can be digested by the enzyme pepsin. HCl also serves to kill a number of pathogens, such as bacteria, viruses, yeast and fungi. Therefore, it is an important defence to stop us getting food poisoning and infections. For example, *E. coli* doesn't survive below a pH of 3.5.

Low hydrochloric acid

There are two main problems that occur when the HCl is insufficient: lack of absorption and decreased capacity to prevent infection.

In the situation of low HCl (hypochloridia) or no HCl (achloridia) the first stages of digestion do not happen properly. If there is not enough acid then also there will be shortages in the production of pepsin. This means that the protein isn't getting broken down efficiently into the individual amino acids. The result is that the body does not receive a sufficient quantity or variety of protein. This can have profound effects on one's health and wellbeing. The body makes important brain chemicals such as serotonin and dopamine from protein that needs to be broken down by HCl.

WHAT CAUSES LOW HCL?

As we age, the parietal cells became less efficient at producing HCl. By the time someone is 50 years old the HCl levels usually begin to decline and by their 60s and 70s the majority of people are not producing the levels they were even in their 50s.

There are a number of medications which are prescribed for symptoms of 'indigestion' and gastric reflex, such as 'proton pump inhibitors'. They reduce the production of HCl by the parietal cells. However, the result of taking these is that the stomach acid becomes more alkaline. Instead of it being a pH of 2 to 3 it can be as alkaline as 4 to 5.

Alcohol can cause low HCl, because it can damage the parietal cells. Stress can also interfere with the production of HCl, as can eating in a rush, not chewing sufficiently and drinking liquids during a meal.

Deficiency of certain nutrients, such as zinc, can in itself create HCl production problems. This can cause a cycle of further deficiency.

Other factors that can play a part include consumption of antibiotics, mercury amalgam fillings (see page 15) and a genetic predisposition.

WHAT HAPPENS IF YOU HAVE LOW HCL?

As mentioned, the acid in the stomach enables us to break down foodstuffs, so that they can be properly absorbed. Low HCl commonly causes vitamin and mineral deficiency. Low vitamin

B12 is a particular problem, as low HCl means low intrinsic factor levels. Intrinsic factor is a co-factor produced by the stomach cells that enables vitamin B12 to be absorbed later on in the digestive tract.

HCl protects us from the infiltration of dangerous parasites, yeasts, fungi and bacteria. Therefore, if the pH of the HCl isn't acidic enough we will then be prone to diarrhoea and upset digestion.

Food that is not effectively digested in the stomach puts an added burden on the small intestine and gut. This can cause dysbiosis, a situation where there is an imbalance of bacterial flora. This can give rise to gut permeability syndrome, where the wrong particles of the food begin to get absorbed, creating allergic reactions in the gut. Some research suggests that this is linked to the manifestation of rheumatoid arthritis and other autoimmune disorders (Arrieta, Bistritz and Meddings 2006; Rooney, Jenkins and Buchanan 1990).

Low HCl also results in some degree of malnutrition, such as deficiency of:

- B vitamins, especially B12

- minerals such as iron, zinc, magnesium, calcium and copper

- protein.

It also results in all manner of symptoms and problems, such as:

- acne rosacea

- eczema and skin conditions

- feeling of excessive fullness after you eat

- increasing number of food sensitivities and allergies

- persistent yeast infections, especially those triggered after eating yeast

- problems with appetite, excessive or lack of appetite
- quick onset of bloating upon eating
- regular feeling of nausea after eating
- thread veins on the face
- unexplained hair loss and thinning
- weak, thin and/or peeling finger nails
- unexplained anaemia
- underweight, even though eating enough calories.

Some practitioners have linked low HCl to:

- autoimmune diseases
- arthritis
- chronic fatigue
- degenerative disorders of all kinds
- gut permeability syndrome
- osteoporosis
- susceptibility to infections, such as from yeast, fungi, parasites, bacterial and viral infections.

There are a number of tests available, such as the Heidelberg test, which can monitor your level of HCl, but these can be expensive.

However, the acid test, which is described in the box on the following page, can easily be done at home and I have found it really useful.

THE ACID TEST

First thing in the morning, on an empty stomach, before eating or drinking anything place quarter of a teaspoon of bicarbonate of soda in 250ml of water. Drink the mixture. Then with a stopwatch, time how long it takes to begin belching:

1 to 2 minutes: normal HCl levels.

2 to 3 minutes: normal to slightly low HCl levels.

3 to 5 minutes: hypochloridia, low HCl levels.

5 minutes or more: achloridia, potentially no HCl.

If there is enough hydrochloric acid then you will normally start belching within two minutes. The belching is caused by carbon dioxide gas created by a chemical reaction between the HCl and the bicarbonate of soda.

RESTORING HEALTHY ACID LEVELS

In ancient medicine the 'fire of digestion' is seen as one of the most important factors in maintaining good health. It is an analogy for the overall power of our digestion. In modern language it translates to our HCl, digestive enzymes and the absorption that food undergoes. There are a number of simple ways to help restore the HCl and the vitality of our digestion.

Cider vinegar

This traditional remedy involves taking at least one teaspoon of cider vinegar in 100ml of water, 15 minutes before each meal. This can be increased up to five teaspoons per dose. The pH of cider vinegar is only about 2.5, but it still seems to be helpful. Many people find this does help their digestion, and after a few weeks do better on the acid test.

Lemon juice

This is more within the range that we need at pH 2.2. It is a classic digestive remedy in most places around the world: a squeeze, or juice of a whole lemon, taken in a little water ten minutes before food as a digestive stimulant. Make sure that you swill water around your mouth thoroughly after drinking the citrus juice to protect your tooth enamel.

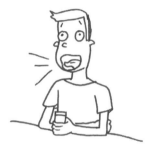

Herbs

Taking herbal bitters can stimulate digestive function. The formula 'Swedish bitters' can be taken before food to promote digestion.

Gentian root tincture, available from a herbalist, can be very helpful. Take ten drops in a little water five to ten minutes before a meal.

Adding black pepper can dramatically increase the absorption of nutrients, as can ingesting fresh ginger in tea and in food on a regular basis.

Digestive teas such as those that contain herbs such as cardamom, ginger, cloves, fennel and cinnamon are excellent for digestion. Drink at least three cups a day.

Regular eating

Our digestive system responds well to a regular routine. Make sure that you eat at least two out of three meals at the same time every day. The most important are your midday meal and not eating too late at night. Sitting down to eat in a relaxed environment is of utmost importance.

Chewing your food thoroughly gives your body a chance to produce sufficient digestive fluids and means it is easier to digest.

Other treatments

Those with a serious deficiency of hydrochloric acid can take a supplement called betaine hydrochloride. However, this is a strong remedy and should be taken only under professional supervision, as too much can cause excess acidity. I have found that gradual changes with food, herbs and supplements usually works well.

Acid indigestion and heartburn

We may think that acid indigestion is caused by too much acid. After all, heartburn is felt around our stomach or oesophagus as acid spills over into the gullet. Ulceration of the stomach can also occur. This can be dangerous as the hydrochloric acid can then cause further destruction of the stomach lining. In serious cases, the acid can digest the stomach wall and spill out into the abdominal cavity, causing peritonitis and even death.

It is now understood that bacteria called *Helicobacter* are responsible for causing stomach ulcers. This doesn't, however, address the underlying cause of the ulcer – and a side-effect of the antibiotic therapy is an imbalance of bacteria in the gut.

The root of the problem is low hydrochloric acid. The correct concentration level would have killed the *Helicobacter pylori* in the first place, thus preventing infestation of the gut. Initially it may seem like a paradox that many people experience relief from acid indigestion by taking an acid substance such as cider vinegar. But if those who regularly experience acid reflux take vinegar preventatively before a meal, they rarely experience symptoms.

Dr Sarah Myhill offers an explanation for acid reflux and the more serious condition of gastro-oesophageal reflux disease (GORD):

> As foods are eaten and enter the stomach, the effect of the food arriving dilutes stomach contents and the acidity rises. The stomach pours in acid to allow digestion of proteins to take place and the pH falls back down to its normal value of 2. The key to understanding GORD is the pyloric sphincter, which is the muscle which controls emptying of the stomach into the duodenum. This muscle is acid sensitive and it only relaxes when the acidity of the stomach is correct, i.e. 2–4. At this point stomach contents can pass into the duodenum (where they are neutralised by bicarbonate released in dribs and drabs from the bile ducts).
>
> If the stomach does not produce enough acid and the pH is only say 5, then the muscle which allows the stomach to empty (the pyloric sphincter) will not open up (dilate). When the stomach contracts in order to move food into the duodenum, the progress of the food is blocked by this contracted pyloric sphincter. But of course the pressure in the stomach increases and the food gets squirted back up into the oesophagus. Although this food is not very acid (not acid enough to relax the pyloric sphincter), it is certainly acid enough to burn the oesophagus and so one gets the symptoms of gastro-oesophageal reflux. The paradox is that this symptom is caused by not enough stomach acid! i.e. the reverse of what is generally believed! (Myhill 2009)

In cases of acid reflux, food sensitivities should be investigated. It is worth trying to eliminate dairy or gluten to see if that helps.

If someone has experienced prolonged episodes of acid reflux then the tissues of the oesophagus may be inflamed and damaged. An endoscopy will reveal what damage has been done, the level of inflammation and whether there are cancerous tissue changes as a result of prolonged acid exposure. Natural solutions for inflammation of the stomach and oesophagus where there is not malignancy include:

- aloe vera gel

- mastic gum

- slippery elm inner bark.

Intestinal dysbiosis

We have a huge variety of bacteria in our digestive tract. There is a delicate symbiotic balance between the different species of micro-flora present in the intestinal tract.

The gastro-intestinal tract is estimated to hold some 100,000 billion bacteria. On average 30 per cent of our stools' mass actually consists of bacteria. It is not known exactly how many different species our gut contains. The Human Microbiome Project was set up in the US in 2008 to discover just how many bacteria the human body contains. At the moment it is estimated that there are between 300 and 1000 species (Sears 2006).

When the bacteria become out of balance then a situation of dysbiosis occurs. Unwanted bacteria and yeasts can get to a state of overgrowth, the most well known in naturopathic circles being Candida.

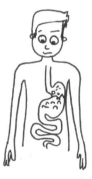

Candida is a species of yeast, one of many fungi. There are many types of Candida, *Candida albicans* being the most common in the human body. Other types are *C. glabrata* and *C. parapsilosis*. In this chapter I will refer to all strains collectively as Candida.

Candida is naturally present in the gut in small quantities, but various factors can cause it to multiply rapidly, causing an assortment of symptoms. Approximately half of my patients are affected by Candida overgrowth or dysbiosis and get relief from a multitude of different conditions when this is treated. Parasitic infections are also frequently found in those who have an overgrowth of yeast.

Ordinarily the gut, using complex processes, will keep yeasts, fungus and unhealthy bacteria under control. Good bacteria help to maintain the balance of the gut ecology, acting as the police force in the digestive tract and preventing unruly infections from taking over. *Lactobacillus acidophilus* and *Bifidum bacterium* are examples of good bacteria.

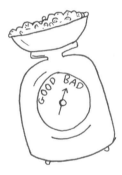

When there is a state of dysbiosis and certain bacteria and yeasts are at a disproportionate level the gut struggles to deal with the toxins that they produce. These include acetaldehyde and ethanol. Acetaldehyde increases the toxic load massively by impairing the healthy functioning of red blood cells (lymphocytes) and interfering with neurotransmitters in the brain. This can result in feeling poisoned, drowsy and fatigued. Acetaldehyde also 'jams up' some of the detox pathways of the liver, predisposing an individual to 'multiple chemical sensitivity'. This manifests itself where there is exposure to small amounts of chemicals, such as strong odours from paint fumes, and can cause internal inflammation and an array of other symptoms. Ethanol can create neurological and psychiatric problems and induce a feeling of having drunk too much alcohol. I have found hidden fungal infections present with most diseases.

When there is a state of dysbiosis and/or yeast overgrowth over a prolonged period of time the gut lining becomes compromised. This causes what is known as gut permeability syndrome, or 'leaky gut', which allows waste products and undigested food such as proteins deeper into the gut mucosa and to enter the bloodstream.

This in turn triggers the immune system into action, causing inflammation, excess mucous production and other symptoms associated with dysbiosis. Next, the liver, which is responsible for handling waste products from the bloodstream, becomes overworked and congested. This further compromises the digestive process, allowing a ready supply of undigested starches and sugars – a food supply for further unwanted bacterial and yeast overgrowth – to develop. A vicious cycle, that is hard to break, has begun.

Symptoms of dysbiosis include:

- abdominal bloating

- abdominal pain

- aches in joints

- alcohol intolerance

- anal itching

- bladder infections

- colitis

- cystitis

- depression

- digestive disturbances

- dry, itchy skin

- excess flatulence
- fatigue
- frequent infections
- foggy brain
- food intolerances
- frequent sore throats
- fungal infections of nail or skin
- headaches
- hormonal irregularities
- IBS (irritable bowel syndrome)
- increased allergies
- joint swelling
- mood swings
- muscle aches
- muscle pain
- PMT (pre-menstrual tension)
- skin problems
- sugar cravings
- frequent episodes of thrush
- weight fluctuation
- white coating on the tongue.

Causes of dysbiosis include:

- antibiotic use
- contraceptive pill, hormone replacement therapy (HRT) and steroids

- diet high in refined carbohydrates and sugar
- immune suppressant drugs and weakened immunity
- insufficient hydrochloric acid in the stomach
- mercury fillings
- pancreatic enzyme deficiency
- prolonged stress.

Gut permeability syndrome can in addition be caused by:

- environmental chemicals
- history of infection from:
    - amoebic dysentery
    - giardia
    - *Salmonella*
- parasites
- pharmaceutical drugs, especially:
    - antibiotics
    - non-steroidal anti-inflammatory drugs (NSAIDS)
    - steroids
- poor diet, alcohol, sugar
- stress.

ANTIBIOTICS

Antibiotics are some of the most frequently prescribed drugs. In certain situations they save lives and they have certainly changed the face of medicine in the twentieth century. However, they should be used sparingly and reserved for serious and life-threatening situations only. Frequent and avoidable use of antibiotics can create a chain of events resulting in immune problems, multiple food sensitivities and chronic fatigue.

Strains of bacteria resistant to antibiotics are now becoming common. A recent study has revealed that, despite warnings from medical authorities, antibiotics are still being over-prescribed, most notably for conditions such as sore throats, ear infections, upper respiratory tract infections and sinusitis (Petersen and Hayward 2007).

Most antibiotics that are prescribed are broad spectrum, that is they do not discriminate in what bacteria they kill. So, during a course of antibiotics many of the friendly bacteria are also destroyed. This leaves a problem in the gut ecology where the yeasts and bad bacteria can no longer be controlled and quickly multiply and overgrow. Even though you may not be taking medically prescribed antibiotics, if you are eating meat and dairy, you probably are ingesting them. Commercially reared animals receive a low dose of antibiotics in their feed to stop them getting infections. Eating commercially produced dairy, meat and eggs exposes you to these antibiotics and hormone residue.

SYNTHETIC HORMONES AND STEROIDS

The contraceptive pill and hormone replacement therapy create an internal cellular environment that predisposes women to yeast infections. Scientists aren't clear why this happens, but believe that the synthetic hormones in the drug affect the detoxification pathways. Steroids suppress the immune system and it is known that steroid inhalers can cause oral thrush or Candida.

DIGESTIVE WEAKNESS

As I have discussed, having the correct amount of hydrochloric acid in the body is essential for digestive health. A lack of 'digestive fire', where there are not sufficient enzymes to break down food, and a diet high in sugar predispose the body to yeast overgrowth.

MERCURY FILLINGS

Mercury disturbs the internal gut ecology. It also suppresses the immune system and upsets cellular respiration. I have seen patients go on restricted diets for years as they battle against overgrowth, only to resolve the problem once they have had their fillings removed.

'DAMP'

In Chinese medicine, they don't use the term dysbiosis or an overgrowth of yeast. Instead, they call this imbalance an invasion of 'damp'. This is essentially a different term for the same symptoms, which include heavy limbs, loose stools, bloating, weight gain, muzzy-headedness and a tendency to worry excessively. In humid conditions, it often makes the patient feel drained and heavy.

Chinese medicine stresses the importance of living in a damp-free environment. It can be difficult to resolve dysbiosis and yeast overgrowth if you live in a damp home. Dehumidifiers, however, can really help.

Simply restricting sugar intake, without using probiotics and antifungals, does not usually result in a permanent rebalancing of the gut flora. What is needed is:

- strict diet change to promote the correct balance of bacteria

- antifungal medicine to kill off all yeasts and unwanted bacteria

- restoration of beneficial bacteria

- improving the detox pathways and restoration of digestive health.

DIET FOR CHRONIC DYSBIOSIS AND LEAKY GUT

First, and most important, remove all sugar from your diet.

Patients are sometimes shocked when faced with what seems like a radical change in their diet. Many say, 'But there is nothing left to eat!' However, by focusing on the many foods that can be eaten on this regime, and by being well organised, you will succeed.

You will quickly adjust to your new regime and, as you start to reap the benefits, find it far less of an inconvenience. Most people notice improvements in the first month, though it can take several months to completely balance the bacteria levels and normalise yeast levels.

Foods to avoid

- *Wheat.* This is a common sensitivity and most people with dysbiosis will need to avoid it. It is in pasta (durum wheat), regular wheat bread and in many other foods, including soups. Check food labels carefully when shopping.

- *Dairy.* Cheese and milk. Many people can tolerate yoghurt and butter.

- *Fruit juices.* This means all types, including canned, bottled or frozen.

- *Alcohol.* If you're cleansing, you'll need all the help your liver can give you.

- *Fresh fruit for the first two to four weeks.* In most cases, fruit needs to be avoided until the yeast is under control. After a month, you can usually introduce one to two pieces of fruit each day.

- *Edible fungi.* All types of mushrooms, morels and truffles.

- *Yeast.* Brewer's yeast, baker's yeast, vitamins and minerals containing yeast, except non-active Engevita yeast.

- *Sugar.* This means anything ending in 'ose' – maltose, dextrose, lactose, sucrose, fructose...you get the idea. They may be hidden away in some foods such as sucrose, glycogen, mannitol, monosaccharides, polysaccharides and sorbitol. Avoid all types of syrup such as maple syrup, golden syrup, molasses, rice syrup, date sugar and, of course...regular sugar.

- *All dried fruits.* Raisins, apricots, dates, prunes, figs and pineapple.

Quite a list, I hear you say. But remember, the yeast could be considered as a parasite. If it is not starved and killed, it will simply return, stronger. That hunger pang, or need for sugar, that you're feeling is the yeast shouting, 'Feed me!'

What you can eat

With food intolerances on the rise, a wider range of alternatives are becoming available in health food shops and supermarkets. So, as I mentioned earlier, organisation is key here. Having the right food available when hunger strikes will keep you on track in the fight against yeast overgrowth and dysbiois. Keeping this list close to your shopping list will help you stock the right foods.

WHEAT ALTERNATIVES

There are many alternatives to wheat, including a huge choice of grains and flours such as corn, millet, quinoa, buckwheat and rice.

- *Pasta.* Wheat-free pastas made from corn, buckwheat, rice and vegetables are available at most supermarkets.

- *Bread.* Rice cakes, corn crackers and Ryvita are ideal substitutes for bread.

- *Noodles.* Rice noodles and buckwheat noodles are fine.

DAIRY ALTERNATIVES

- *Milk.* Oat milk and almond milk. (Milk that has had the lactose removed can still be a problem.)

- *Butter.* There are dairy-free spreads such as 'Pure', although I am not a big fan of margarine. Humus or tahini make good spreads, although most people can tolerate dairy in the form of butter.

- *Cheese.* Sorry, but there are no alternatives to cheese. I believe soya cheese is highly processed junk.

- *Sugar.* Anything that tastes sweet is going to be high on the glycaemic index. Artificial sweeteners such as aspartame are not suitable for detoxification and are potentially toxic. There is a type of sugar called Xylitol, though its qualities are currently unproven. Early indications are that it might be suitable for those with yeast overgrowth.

- *Condiments.* Herbs and spices are excellent for adding flavour to food. You can also use tamari or Braggs Aminos soya sauce, both of which are wheat-free. Olives are great with many types of food and sundried tomatoes can really help too. Try them with avocado and humus on Ryvita. (See also Cousins 2000a, 2000b.)

- *Meat, eggs and fish.* Organic meat, eggs and fish do not need to be restricted to reduce Candida. However, red meat should not be consumed on any kind of diet regime. If you find red meat too difficult to cut from your diet, try reducing your intake to once or twice a week. When moving over to a detox vegetarian diet, organic fish can help you make the transition.

Useful remedies

There are a number of medicines that can be taken for yeast, bacterial overgrowth and dysbiosis. Here are some of the options that I have found to work particularly well.

- *Caprylic acid.* Derived from coconuts, caprylic acid is an antifungal, antibacterial fatty acid that promotes good bacteria. It is naturally present in breast milk, which is why breastfed babies are less likely to suffer from thrush than those fed from the bottle. Caprylic acid is not recommended if there is inflammatory disease of the gut such as colitis.

- *Grapefruit seed extract.* An antifungal and antimicrobial agent 'par excellence', grapefruit seed extract has antiparasitic qualities and works well with caprylic acid. It is available in liquid form, which is good for a systemic effect, but reaches the yeast in the gut best when taken in capsule form. It is not suitable for patients taking warfarin. In my clinic, I use a combined version called Caprylic Complex.

- *Horopito and aniseed.* Horopito (*Pseudowintera colorata*) was traditionally taken by the Maori people of New Zealand for digestive complaints. Combined with aniseed it has a synergistic affect, is highly antifungal and usually well tolerated when the gut is inflamed.

- *Oregano (Origanum vulgare).* This common culinary herb has many antibacterial and antifungal qualities. Freeze-dried oil in capsules works well, especially combined with grapefruit seed extract.

- *Myrrh (Commiphora molmol).* Prized over centuries for its remarkable healing characteristics, myrrh is a tree resin containing medicinal volatile oils. It is also antimicrobial. I use this in capsules, though the tincture form can be gargled to treat oral thrush. Myrrh also has anti-inflammatory actions and boosts the number of white blood cells.

DYSBIOSIS PROGRAMME

A typical dysbiosis programme would be:

Week 1
Make a shift in your diet, but do it gradually over a week.

Weeks 2–4
Begin taking antifungals such as myrrh (two capsules before breakfast and a further two before your evening meal) and probiotics (two capsules after breakfast and two after your evening meal). Continue with the antifungals for one month.

Week 5
Change to a different type of antifungal, such as Caprylic Complex. Take two capsules in the morning before breakfast and a further two before your evening meal. Keep taking the probiotics as usual.

The reason for varying the antifungal is that Candida can develop a resistance to any one type if taken continuously. Expect it to take at least two to three months to get the yeast back under control. You will also notice a change in your general health and bowel movements.

Beneficial bacteria

High strength, potent probiotics are essential. They should contain a full spectrum of good bacteria, including *L. acidophilus*, *L. plantarum*, *L. bulgaricus*, *L. rhamnosus* and *B. bifidum*. Unfortunately, the varieties sold in health food shops are rarely potent enough, and yoghurt, while rich in probiotics, is not rich enough. You would have to drink several litres of yoghurt to match the quantity of probiotics in a single clinical strength capsule. As a guide, a capsule should have a minimum of 4 billion bacteria to be medicinally useful.

Side-effects

As the unwanted bacteria and yeasts are controlled, die-off reactions are not uncommon. When yeast is being killed off, it tries to fight back. Levels of toxins such as acetaldehyde, which the Candida excretes, often increase when targeted by the detox process. At this stage, people may experience symptoms such as headaches, bloating, wind, feeling 'spacey' and generally unwell. This is a normal part of the process but it shouldn't last too long. A few days of feeling slightly unwell is the average.

As with all detoxification programmes, if you have several symptoms, or a complicated health picture, it would be wise to be under the supervision of a practitioner experienced in working with gut detoxification and restoration.

Leaky gut

The intestinal lining, called the gut mucosa, and the good bacteria in the digestive tract are designed to recognise 'friend from foe'. This ensures that only nutrients such as fats, starches and proteins get absorbed into the bloodstream.

Dysbiosis, the bacterial imbalance or disturbed ecology of the gut, can occur as a result of infections or the taking of medical drugs. This creates an environment in which foreign infections such as yeast overgrowth (Candida), *Helicobacter pylori*, *Blastocystis hominis*, amoebas, *Salmonella*, parasites and others can grow.

Common culprits for killing beneficial bacteria include antibiotics, non-steroidal anti-inflammatory drugs (NSAIDs), the contraceptive pill, steroids, chemotherapy and radiotherapy. Heavy metals, especially mercury from amalgam fillings, are also implicated.

FOOD SENSITIVITY

When the lining of the gut becomes inflamed and compromised it can give rise to food allergies and sensitivities. Food sensitivities may occur as a chain of immune reactions are triggered when eating certain foods. Allowed to continue, these food sensitivities often worsen. Many times I have seen people who have avoided foods for an extended period of time while the underlying problem has remained untreated. The effect is increased sensitivity to more and more foods.

It is possible to test for leaky gut with a gut permeability test. This can determine how 'leaky' the gut is. It is possible that someone no longer has a state of dysbiosis, but that the body has not been able to repair the situation. Therefore it is still possible to have symptoms such as:

- abdominal pain

- acne

- anxiety

- arthritis

- autoimmune diseases

- bloating

- chronic fatigue

- constipation

- diarrhoea

- food sensitivities

- inflammatory bowel diseases such as Crohn's disease

- irritable bowel

- psoriasis

- tiredness after eating

- wind.

The involvement of leaky gut in disease has been the subject of a number of medical papers. Coverage of autoimmune diseases, where the body's immune system attacks itself, is especially prevalent among this writing. One reason for this is that, with leaky gut, substances are present in the body that shouldn't be. As a result, inappropriate immune processes are taking place to protect the body.

HEALING THE HOLES

There are a number of nutritional and botanical remedies that can promote the healing of the gut lining:

- Butyric acid is a short chain fatty acid that feeds the epithelial mucosa cells lining the gut wall. It is available in capsule form and usually needs to be used for at least six months.

- Medicinal clay such as bentonite can be taken and can promote gut repair and detoxification. One teaspoon in water three times a day promotes gut detoxification and repair.

NATURAL MEDICINE AND THE GUT

Holistic understanding of the gut

In Chinese and Ayurvedic medicine, digestion is considered central to the health of the whole body. And good digestion begins with good food. However, the quality of food lies in more than its mere nutritional content. The qi – energy contained in the food – is also influenced by the thoughts and emotions of the cook. To get an idea of this concept, think of how much you enjoy a meal cooked with love compared with one prepared in a rush. This is an important principle in ancient medicine. In Ayurvedic cooking the cook is not permitted to taste the food during preparation. It is to be created as a sacred offering to the divine.

Gut feeling

Our ability to think is related to digestion. This is because almost all substances that direct the brain's functions, such as serotonin and dopamine, can be found in the gut. An imbalance in the gut will affect the brain and vice versa. This is why stress and emotional upsets affect our bowel movements and digestion. It also means that disturbances in the gut will have an impact on our brain chemistry and the way we think.

In Chinese medicine the ability to think is centred around our digestive organs. The capacity to take on new ideas is directly related to the strength of our stomachs and the health of our digestive systems.

As we saw earlier, the small intestine sorts the pure from the impure. And this applies just as much to concepts and ideas as it does to physical digestion.

Many of us go through periods when we eat poorly – and they usually coincide with periods of intense mental exertion. When I was training as an acupuncturist, I knew well that eating a healthy diet when studying would be the best plan, but I craved foods such as sugar and pizzas. When we think excessively, we weaken our digestive powers. And from that imbalance comes the craving for foods that take us further out of sync. Then, when our physical digestion is weak we have difficulties in digesting thoughts and concepts: we get brain fog and have a tendency to obsessive thoughts.

To redress the balance of our digestion, it is necessary to cleanse the gut of toxins and restore its vitality.

The large intestine – the drainer of the dregs – eliminates the toxins from the body. This, as has been understood in all traditions for thousands of years, helps us let go of emotions as well. The idea that someone is anally retentive, reintroduced by Freud at the start of the twentieth century and suggesting that person is overly fussy and controlling, bears this out.

HEALING THE DIGESTION

The keys to healing an upset digestion system are:

- restoring healthy levels of hydrochloric acid and digestive enzymes by reigniting the digestive fire

- restoring healthy liver function

- avoiding foods detrimental to digestive health and eating foods with correct levels of fibre

- resolving dysbiosis and killing harmful yeast overgrowth

- having healthy elimination and bowel movements to get the waste out

- consuming healthy bacteria such as in fermented foods.

Relight my fire

'Digestive fire' is a term used in ancient medicines to summarise the body's ability to break down and absorb nutrition from our food. It encompasses everything from adequate hydrochloric acid levels in the stomach, through sufficient breakdown of enzymes, to the absorption of nutrition into the bloodstream.

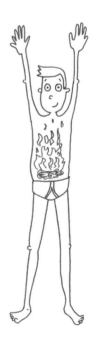

Some factors, however, can dampen the digestive fire. A cloying mucous-like substance can attach to the small intestine and prevent us metabolising our food properly. In Ayurveda they call this ama, while in Chinese medicine it is called damp. Both terms are alternative ways of describing conditions such as Candida, yeast overgrowth, dysbiosis and leaky gut.

You know you have good digestion when:

- you feel comfortable after eating

- you have bowel movements at least once a day

- your stools are free of blood, mucous and undigested food and are easy to pass

- you pass little or no wind with only slight or no odour.

SECRET RECIPE FOR A TOP DIGESTIVE SYSTEM

2 tsp organic goat yogurt

8 tsp mineral water

15 cardamom seeds – crushed

1 cinnamon stick (1 inch long) crushed

1 whole red onion, chopped and blended

½ cup pomegranate juice

Mix the ingredients into a thick drink and consume at mid-morning and/or afternoon for three days. This can be repeated once a week for up to a month to improve the overall digestion, increase absorption and stimulate the production of digestive juices and enzymes.

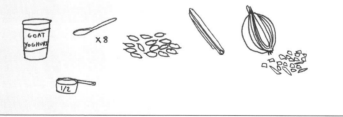

GUIDELINES FOR GOOD DIGESTIVE HEALTH

Eating and drinking

- *Chew* your food thoroughly. This is an all-important first stage in digestion and one that most of us don't take enough time over. As they say, the stomach does not have teeth!

- *Avoid drinking liquids* when eating – this dilutes the digestive juices.

- *Sit down* when you eat.

- *Don't mix fruit* with other foods. Eat fruit at least one hour before or after other foods. Fruit ferments in the gut when eaten too close to other foods.

- *Don't eat late at night.* This results in incomplete digestion of food and can contribute towards insomnia and waking up feeling sluggish and tired in the morning.

Colon

The colon is responsible for managing and releasing waste in the form of stools, or faeces. The colon is home to a mass of good bacteria that keep harmful bacteria under control.

Diverticular disease is a silent epidemic in the Western world. This occurs when the colon develops a small pouch, also known as a diverticula. These pouches normally contain faecaliths – pieces of faecal matter that get trapped on their way out of the body – in mini-herniations. These small sacs full of old decaying matter are, potentially, hugely toxic. When they become infected, and inflamed, diverticulitis results.

Some health professionals believe that diverticular disease is caused by constipation and is found only among people in the developed world. It doesn't occur in tribal peoples, or those with high-fibre diets.

Food transit time

Regardless of how healthily we eat, if our food is not digested properly and the waste evacuated completely, we can still have big problems.

Bowel movements should be regular and frequent – once or twice each day. Studies of indigenous peoples have revealed that they have a bowel movement for each meal they consume.

If the transit time is too short, vital nutrition from the food will not have been absorbed. If it is too long, putrefaction will take place. Food reaches a temperature of 37°C in the gut – the temperature of an extremely hot sunny day. Average transit time is 24 hours, but 48 to 72 hours is relatively common, which means that food can be 'digesting' in a very hot place for three days. In short, it is decomposing and rotting in the gut. Naturally forming toxins will then spill over from the gut into the rest of the body, creating autotoxaemia, a process of self-poisoning.

I treat many children with constipation. I have seen many that struggle to have a bowel movement every ten days. Then, when they do, it is so big and hard that it causes rectal bleeding and pain. They often have fevers, which are treated with antibiotics or paracetamol. However, because the fever originates from infected waste matter that has been in the body for too long, it will subside once a pattern of regular bowel movements is established. Ingesting probiotics is completely essential, as is restricting foods that they might be allergic to.

BOWEL CLEANSE FORMULA

Bowel detoxification can be further stimulated by the ingestion of the bowel cleanse powder, made from equal parts of the following:

activated charcoal

apple fruit pectin

bentonite clay

psyllium husks

slippery elm inner bark

I use a formula based on all these five ingredients in my clinic to promote detoxification of chemicals, heavy metals and radioactivity. I usually prescribe at least one teaspoon of this mixture a minimum of three times daily. It is vitally important that you continue to have regular bowel movements while ingesting this, in order for the toxins to get out. Drinking prune juice, or soaking a tablespoon of linseeds in water left overnight and the whole mixture drunk in the morning, normally does the trick. Drinking the linseed mixture is very helpful for chronic constipation. Herbal laxatives containing Senna pods or Cascara Sagrada should only be used in an emergency and for a maximum of a couple of weeks.

HOW DO I MAKE THE BOWEL CLEANSE FORMULA?

You should mix the bowel cleanse powder in a jam jar with water/apple juice, shake it and drink it immediately. It is important to ensure that at least a litre of water is drunk throughout the day.

Chapter 5

ELIMINATION/ DETOXIFICATION

Diseases are crises of purification, of toxic elimination.
(Hippocrates, 450 BC)

WHAT ARE TOXINS?

Toxins are the waste products of a healthy and properly functioning body. We eat, we assimilate and we produce waste. There are two types of toxins, exogenous and endogenous.

Exogenous toxins – from the environment

Exogenous toxins originate outside of the body, such as bacteria and viruses, as well as some of the environmental toxins discussed in previous chapters.

Endogenous toxins – created from within

Metabolic waste is created as part of our normal and healthy existence. For example, we inhale oxygen and exhale carbon dioxide. When we digest and process protein, we create nitrogenous wastes such as uric acid, urea and ammonia. These are processes that enable us to function.

Sometimes these endogenous toxins can become too much for the body to deal with, and some degree of autointoxication occurs. A common area is the teeth and gums. A periodontal pocket can develop between the gum and the teeth, and provide a breeding ground for bacteria. A toxic load can then build up, increasing the risk of stroke and heart attacks: 'Those with gum disease are almost twice as likely to suffer from coronary artery disease' (American Academy of Periodontology 2011).

The gut itself contains a multitude of beneficial bacteria, most of which are benign and essential. There are others, such as yeast and fungus, that release toxins in our system in the form of aldehyde and alcohol.

Ancient medical systems such as Ayurveda recognise that there are times when the body can get overwhelmed with its own metabolic toxins. When this happens our natural processes become impaired, leaving us vulnerable to disease.

ENEMAS

Raising the subject of enemas with patients usually results in a deathly silence. Historically, however, the enema has been of great medicinal benefit in most cultures.

At the Vatican, there is an ancient Aramaic text called the Essene Gospel of Peace. It clearly extols the virtues of the enema:

> Seek, therefore, a large trailing gourd, having a stalk the length of a man; take out its contents and fill it with water from the river which the sun has warmed up. Hang it upon the branch of a tree, and kneel upon the ground before the angel of water, and suffer the end of the stalk of the trailing gourd to enter your hinder parts that the water may flow through all of your bowels. Afterwards rest kneeling on the ground before the angel of water and pray to the living God that he will free your body from every un-cleanliness and disease. Then let the water run out of your body, that it may carry within it all the unclean and evil-smelling things...
> (Szekely 1981)

In Ayurveda, enemas are used not just for cleansing but also to introduce medicinal substances such as herbs, ghee and honey into the body. These substances are used to encourage healing, particularly among the weak and malnourished.

Enemas are an excellent way to bring a fever down as they help to stimulate the removal of toxins. Fever is often accompanied by constipation, which in turn can cause temperature to rise further. Acting as a purgative, an enema can break the cycle.

Herbal enemas can reduce inflammation. One such type of enema is called a rectal syringe (it sounds more gruesome than it is). This is a bulb with a nozzle that allows viscous liquids such as fresh aloe vera juice, flaxseed tea and oils to be released into the bowel. This is usually recommended for inflammatory bowel conditions.

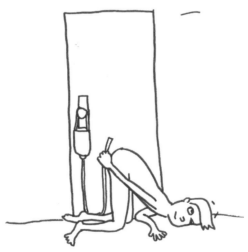

Enemas for detoxification

For the purpose of detoxification, I am going to discuss how to perform an enema using water, herbal teas or coffee.

Note: Liquids should always be strained through a muslin cloth whenever a non-water ingredient is used.

How to take an enema

You will need:

gravity bag enema kit

thermometer

olive oil

1 litre of one of the following: filtered water; herbal tea; coffee decoction

The ideal place to do the enema is a warm bathroom.

1. If using a non-water ingredient, strain the liquid through a muslin cloth and allow to cool.

2. Hang the enema bag on the back of the door handle. If you place it too high it can be a little too forceful. Make sure the tap is turned off or the clamp near the nozzle is shut. The liquid must be at body temperature (37°C/98.4°F) – use the thermometer to check. It should feel barely warm to the touch. Fill the bag carefully with the liquid. As there will be some air in the tube, open the tap and let the liquid flow into the toilet or sink. Once the air has gone, turn off the tap or close the clamp.

3. Next, place a large towel on the floor, then lubricate the tip of the tube with olive oil. For water and herb tea enemas, begin the procedure by lying on your left-hand side. For coffee enemas, lie on your right-hand side for the entire process.

4. Draw your legs up towards your chest and breathe slowly. Now, carefully insert the lubricated tip of the tube into your anus. Keep breathing slowly, take your time and relax.

5. Turn on the tap and allow the fluid to flow into your rectum. At this point during a water or herbal tea enema, you can move onto your back. You may find you can absorb more liquid by then rolling onto your right-hand side.

6. After all of the liquid (or as much as you can take) has drained into the bowel, turn off the tap and carefully remove the tip from your anus. For maximum medicinal effect try to retain the mixture, relax, keep warm and stay lying down for at least ten minutes.

7. When you're done, stand up slowly. You may feel a little light-headed at this stage – don't worry, this is normal. Finally, release your bowels on the toilet.

WATER

The simplest enema to perform uses plain filtered water, slightly warmed. Introducing water into the rectum can encourage the emptying of the bowel, so this form is good for occasional constipation or for cleansing to facilitate further elimination.

HERBAL TEAS

Herbal teas, used instead of water, provide extra medicinal benefit. Chamomile tea promotes relaxation and reduces spasms. Fenugreek tea can reduce pain such as that experienced by people with the digestive disease diverticulitis.

COFFEE

Coffee has some amazing detoxifying properties which stimulate numerous cleansing chain reactions in the body. Drinking it, however, does not produce these effects. To get the benefits of coffee, we have to take it rectally.

Coffee enemas reportedly originated in German hospitals during World War I. When supplies of painkillers, particularly those for post-operative care, ran very low, enemas were used commonly to aid recovery. To help with the pain, soldiers were often given coffee to drink. Somehow, when administered in an enema it was noted as being much more useful for pain relief and supporting recovery than water.

In the 1920s, research was carried out at the Goettingen College of Medicine into this seemingly bizarre discovery. The scientists found that caffeinated enemas, administered to rats, stimulated the opening of the liver's bile ducts.

Dr Max Gerson was the first clinician to use coffee enemas for detoxification purposes as part of the Gerson cancer therapy in the 1930s (see Gerson 1990). Subsequent research supported the effects of his work.

Once introduced into the rectum, theophylline and theobromine in the coffee cause the blood vessels in the bowel and the bile ducts to dilate. The coffee is absorbed through the mesenteric vein and carried to the liver by the portal vein. This causes a dumping of bile and toxins from the liver and bloodstream into the small intestine.

Coffee enemas have a powerful detoxification effect. It is believed that, when taken rectally, the palmatic acids contained in the coffee massively enhance the enzyme glutathione S-transferase (GST). This is part of the body's strongest natural antioxidant delivering system and is vital for Phase I and II of the detoxification pathways (see page 149). As mentioned in the section on the liver (see page 146), glutathione is probably the main ingredient needed for our body to detoxify correctly.

The coffee enema

Add three tablespoons of organic ground coffee to one litre of filtered water. (Do not use instant coffee powder or granules – instant coffee is not suitable for an enema.)

Boil the coffee/water mix for two to three minutes and then simmer for 20 minutes. Strain through a muslin cloth and allow to cool to body temperature (37°C/98.4°F) – use the thermometer to check. It should feel barely warm to the touch. Pour all of the mixture into the enema bag.

Once in the bowel, the coffee should remain in place for approximately 15 minutes. The body's entire blood supply is filtered through the liver every three to four minutes. After a 15-minute coffee enema, the blood is efficiently detoxified and blood serum toxin levels are significantly reduced.

Enemas for dry bowel movements

If you have very dry bowel movements, avoid plain water enemas as they may further dry your bowel. Instead, opt for mucilaginous (moist and sticky) herbs as these help to rehydrate and moisturise the tissues. Add a tablespoon of fenugreek seeds or flaxseeds to a litre of water and simmer for ten minutes.

Strain the fluids through a muslin cloth before using.

When not to take an enema

Unless given under professional supervision, enemas should be avoided if you have any bowel condition, rectal bleeding or high blood pressure. Enemas are also not advised for pregnant women, the very ill or the weak.

Enemas on children should also be avoided unless provided under professional supervision. They are, however, very effective in bringing down a fever in a child.

Enemas taken under the direction of a qualified practitioner can encourage detoxification; however, they should not be relied upon to stimulate bowel movements outside of a cleansing regime. Long-term use of enemas could create a dependency and weaken the bowel. Coffee enemas can be contraindicated for those who are currently on, or have at any time received, chemotherapy or medical drugs, as residues of the drugs can be released into the bloodstream and potentially cause toxicity. They can also be contraindicated for alcoholics, diabetics, substance users, those with neurological conditions and pregnant women.

Chapter 6

FANTASTIC FASTING

Instead of using medicine, rather, fast a day. (Plutarch, AD 46–120)

Everyone has a physician inside him or her; we just have to help it in its work. The natural healing force within each one of us is the greatest force in getting well. Our food should be our medicine. Our medicine should be our food. But to eat when you are sick is to feed your sickness. (Hippocrates, 460–370 BC)

In the Western world, fasting was reintroduced as a medical technique in the early 1800s by doctors such as Isaac Jennings in the USA and Father Kneipp in Germany. By the beginning of the twentieth century, naturopathic medicine was well established: John Harvey Kellogg, who famously invented the cornflakes breakfast cereal, also ran the Battle Creek Sanatorium where he would have up to a thousand people fasting at a time.

Naturopath Bernard Jensen also became inspired by the benefits of fasting. Jensen practised iridology (the study of the human iris) and its relationship with certain constitutional types of iris patterning. He travelled around the world searching for the healthiest indigenous cultures. He realised that in most cultures fasting was often undertaken routinely, or was practised when people were ill. Through clinical experience, and by tailoring his nature cure programmes for different types of iris patterns, he found he could further improve the effects of clinical fasting in relation to a body's inherent resistance as seen in the patient's iris.

Teachers of mine, herbalists Kitty Campion and Richard Schulze, were major proponents of fasting, having recommended 'juice fasting' to thousands of their patients. Both were inspired by their training with the eclectic herbalist Dr John Christopher.

WHAT IS FASTING?

A fast is the avoidance of all or the majority of foods. There are different types of fast; some involve drinking just water or juices, while others are mono fast, involving eating just one type of food such as grapes for a predetermined number of days. Fasting is probably the most ancient of all self-healing techniques.

To our modern minds, it may seem illogical that avoiding food can assist anything but weight loss. However, done in the right way, fasting can be one of the most powerful self-healing options available to us. All ancient systems of medicine include fasting as part of their therapeutic regimes. In ancient Chinese medicine, fasting is an integral part of Taoist spiritual and medical disciplines, usually involving the drinking of water and medicinal teas. Since the communist revolution in China, however, fasting has been actively discouraged because it is linked with Buddhist and Taoist spiritual practices. In Europe the Greek physicians such as Hippocrates and Galen routinely used fasting therapy with their patients.

It is, in fact, difficult to find a culture, apart from modern-day civilisation, in which fasting is not an important healing principle.

In Ayurveda, fasting is classed as 'the first and most important of all medicines'. In this system of medicine, toxins are deemed to originate in the digestive system. Through fasting, these toxins are digested in the body, then broken down and eliminated.

When animals are unwell, they usually stop eating for a few days to aid their recuperation. Most of us, when we are ill, experience loss of appetite. This is our body telling us to rest by not eating.

THE PHYSICAL BENEFITS OF FASTING

As a general principle, when we abstain from food we activate healing processes in the body. In the 1970s my father attended a lecture in California by the famous naturopath, Paul Bragg. Even though Bragg was in his eighties at this time, my father remembers him being a very fit and vital man. In his book, *The Miracle of Fasting*, Paul Bragg wrote:

> Fasting works by self-digestion. During a fast your body intuitively will decompose and burn only the substances and tissues that are damaged, diseased, or unneeded, such as: abscesses, tumours, excess fat deposits, excess water, and congestive wastes. Even a short fast (1 to 3 days) will accelerate elimination from your liver, kidneys, lungs, bloodstream and skin. (Bragg 2004)

Without food to digest, the body goes into a different gear and speeds up the elimination of metabolic waste.

Research in the twentieth century has also demonstrated the benefits of fasting, or the 'fasting cure' – particularly in cases of toxic poisoning where no antidote is available. Sixteen patients poisoned by the ingestion of rice oil contaminated with poly-chlorobiphenyls (PCBs) in Taiwan voluntarily took part in a trial fast, of either seven or ten days' duration. The participants had been poisoned approximately between 26 and 35 months prior to the trial. During fasting, they followed a fixed dietary schedule, consuming mixed juices of fresh vegetables, fruits and boiled soybean. Every patient showed signs of improvements in their poison-related symptoms, some of them dramatic in the relief of severe headache, lumbago, arthritis, cough, mucous and acne eruptions (Imamura and Tung 1984).

Other studies have demonstrated that fasting can promote healthy blood sugar levels in people with diabetes, and reduce the severity and frequency of seizures among people with epilepsy (Allen 1915; Guelpa 1910; Lennox and Cobb 1928). I have seen patients with autoimmune diseases benefit enormously from fasting, particularly those with rheumatoid arthritis. A study in Scandinavia in which patients undertook a fast followed by a vegetarian diet for one year had similar results (Kjeldsen-Kragh *et al.* 1991).

I have also observed improvements in patients with inflammatory bowel conditions such as colitis and Crohn's disease. One patient managed to avert an operation to remove her colon by drinking just carrot juice for ten days. To this day, she remains free of symptoms.

I once dropped a large weight on my right foot, creating a two-inch wound, which then got contaminated by infected water. This developed into septicaemia and I had the fever from hell. Through fasting and the use of a huge amount of Echinacea, however, I managed to cure myself – though not without overdosing on the alcoholic tincture and getting slightly tipsy! It took about three days for the swelling to go down and for the sepsis to resolve. After a week I had made a full recovery.

So, fasting can be beneficial in a number of different cases and, by resting the gut, can promote healing processes that would not otherwise occur. When someone has a disease or health condition it should, however, always be done under close supervision, and serious conditions should be closely monitored by a health professional. In my early days of practice I had a patient who had severe Crohn's disease, which developed into a bowel abscess. Even though we tried natural intervention, the condition deteriorated and, eventually, life-saving surgery was necessary.

FASTING AND MENTAL HEALTH

The benefits of fasting on mental health are also significant. A part of many ancient psychiatric approaches to mental illness, fasting, together with prayer, has also been used for spiritual purposes and has been known to have a stabilising effect on the psyche.

In modern times, too, a number of independent researchers have used fasting to treat mental illness. Dr Yuri Nikolayev, who worked at the Moscow Research Institute of Psychiatry in the 1970s, conducted fasting regimes with over 10,000 people over a 30-year period, during which he demonstrated its value in treating mental illness, particularly schizophrenia (Seeger 1972).

While writing this book I undertook a few fasts to help clear my mind. Like most people who fast, I experienced a change in consciousness and the ability to think more lucidly. This sensation usually comes in waves, with periods of light-headedness alternating with phases of incredible clearness and peace.

EMOTIONAL AND SPIRITUAL ASPECTS OF FASTING

I know many people who report that fasting gives them clarity of thought during periods of confusion or indecision in their lives. This would explain why fasting is encouraged as a spiritual discipline to help us feel more connected with our spiritual selves.

In Islam, Ramadan is a fasting regime. In Christianity there is Lent. Jesus fasted for 40 days and 40 nights. In India there is fasting on the appearance day of Lord Krishna and other saints. In Vaisnavism, an Indian spiritual tradition, every two weeks with the cycle of the moon there is a day called Ekadasi. On this day, people abstain from grains, legumes and pulses. Some devotees go even further and fast from all food to maximise the spiritual benefit. And one day each year there is nir-jal, which is Sanskrit for 'without water'. It is believed that fasting on this day increases one's love and connection to the divine.

When the US Constitution was being drafted, its creators fasted to gain inspiration and clear insight. Abraham Lincoln and George Washington were famous fasters. Perhaps best known of all, however, was Mahatma Gandhi, whose periods of fasting facilitated political reform in his homeland, India.

Fasting can restore equilibrium and sense of self. I have known many people who, after experiencing trauma, have used fasting to get their lives back on track.

My friend and colleague, Muhammed Salim Khan, wrote this in his book on Islamic medicine on the subject of fasting:

> Sawm – complete fasting – is one institution that combines the spiritual, physical, individual and community needs in a most harmonious act. The spiritual aspect of an individual is developed and enhanced in the most sublime manner. Taqwa – God consciousness, discipline and empathy with the poor and needy – are the main emphasis behind fasting. Fasting as a devotional process and internal purification enables the person to transcend his gross and physical needs. The deep cleansing process clears the mind and the internal organs and tissues. Biologically, fasting is an effective, natural process of detoxification and healing. (Khan 1986)

Fasting allows us to review our relationship with food. When changes occur in our emotional state, we often turn to so-called comfort foods – especially sugars and carbohydrates. Fasting can bring emotional issues to light, suggesting that we may be eating to block their impact.

Here, Tracy, a patient of mine, describes her experience of a fast.

Case history: Fasting

'At first it was a bit difficult but after a few days I got really into it. I have battled with being overweight for a number of years and tried lots of diets. When I was just consuming juice and no food I was aware that feelings came up around being lonely. My father died when I was just five and I think I was suppressing the feelings of grief with eating. During the fast I finally disconnected them in my head. I allowed myself to feel sad and didn't block it with eating. Since the fast I consider I have a healthy relationship with food again. I have to catch myself occasionally but my weight is now what it should be.'

FASTING AND FOOD SENSITIVITIES

Another therapeutic aspect to fasting is the suspension of food allergies and sensitivities – most notably when on strict water or mono diets. Very often the relief from the symptoms of such sensitivities is immediate. This is especially true when a food affects the brain and the mental state of a patient without necessarily causing physical symptoms.

I attended a lecture by Canadian psychiatrist Abram Hoffer where he described how he fasted some 200 patients on just water. This had a cleansing effect and eliminated potential food allergens. Then, after four to five days, Dr Hoffer would gradually introduce foods. He noted that some patients would have some kind of relapse immediately after eating the allergen.

One of Dr Hoffer's cases concerned a woman who was schizophrenic, catatonic and unable to walk. After five days of fasting her condition was vastly improved and she was able to walk freely. The fast continued until the patient was completely well. When foods were reintroduced to her diet, the illnesses returned. It was discovered that this woman was allergic to meat, and as long as she avoided it she was fine.

Dr Hoffer called it a brain allergy, which he said was a condition in 60 per cent of his patients. Once these patients stopped consuming the foods they were sensitive to, their conditions either improved or returned to a fully healthy state.

Bizarrely, the foods that people most crave are ones that they are most likely to be allergic to. It is often possible to identify the problem foods by studying a one-week food diary.

At my clinic there have been countless occasions where the avoidance of certain foods has alleviated a multitude of problems – the usual suspects being wheat, cow dairy, eggs and oranges.

It goes without saying that E numbers and artificial sweeteners should be avoided. However, people are often shocked that when they avoid, say, bread, their headaches disappear, or ankle pains that have been plaguing them simply vanish, only to return once the food is eaten again.

Food sensitivities and allergies indicate a leaky gut. Bowel cleansing, the resolution of yeast and dysbiosis and gut repair will sometimes eliminate an allergy, allowing us to enjoy the food in question again without any reaction.

DIFFERENT TYPES OF FAST

Strictly speaking, a fast means eating nothing. However, there are variations on this interpretation and a variety of fasts have been developed over many years to suit the needs of different people. Let's take a look at them.

Mono fast

As its name suggests, a mono fast permits one type of food – and one only. A famous example of this is the grape diet, developed by Dr Joanna Brandt, who had inoperable stomach cancer and, after fasting for five days on water, decided to proceed by eating only grapes, felt better, and continued to eat only grapes until she was cured. Dr Brandt went on to share her discovery with other people, working particularly closely with people with cancer.

Her regime began with a diet of pure water only for the first three days. On the fourth day, a couple of glasses of water upon waking would be followed by grapes. The seeds would be removed but the skins chewed thoroughly. Grapes would continue to be taken every two hours until seven meals of grapes had been consumed. This would be repeated daily for two weeks. In some cases, people would take the grape diet for up to a month. Another feature of Dr Brandt's grape diet was a daily water enema.

I personally don't recommend the grape diet – we are living in a different era and because of the mass use of antibiotics many people suffer from gut dysbiosis and therefore a fast high in sugar, albeit fructose, can be detrimental.

Watermelon fast

I often recommend the watermelon fast to my patients. It is simple and easy to fit into a busy lifestyle. And because it still involves digesting food, it is also ideal for first-time fasters.

Watermelons contain a high concentration of water – about 95 per cent – and are high in potassium, calcium, phosphorus, magnesium, iron, zinc and vitamins A and C. Being very cooling, watermelons are ideal when there is excess heat in the body due to conditions such as a fever, acne and infections or the effects of overexposure to heat, for example sunstroke. They have anti-inflammatory properties. The watermelon fast can also lower blood pressure.

Although the red watermelon flesh is mildly diuretic, the seeds are very stimulating to the kidney and bladder (see the kidney flush on page 195).

Most people find that fasting on watermelon for one to three days is sufficient to give the body a thorough cleansing. Choose ripe, preferably organic, watermelons and be sure to eat plenty of the fruit's flesh and drink at least one litre of water each day.

The watermelon fast is not for people who are thin, anaemic or very cold. Building juices such as beetroot offer these people far greater benefits.

Three-day apple fast

This is a simple cleanse that encourages the elimination of metabolic and environmental toxins and can be helpful when someone has gut permeability (leaky gut syndrome). It is a good alternative to the watermelon fast and usually well tolerated whatever the season. It is recommended by the famous promoter of natural remedies, Edgar Cayce, to 'cleanse all toxic forces from any system' (Reilly and Hagy Brod 2008).

Apples contain pectin, a negatively charged complex polysaccharide, which is able to bind to toxic metals. As a water-soluble fibre it is able to pass through the digestive tract and draw out exogenous toxins. It was discovered that when apple pectin was added to the diet of people residing in areas affected by radiation from Chernobyl, it effectively and significantly encouraged the excretion of radioactive caesium-137 (Yablokov 2009).

HOW TO DO THE APPLE FAST

On each day, eat as many apples as you feel comfortable with. Most people eat a minimum of five in the day. It is important that the apples are organic and if possible a mixture of varieties. When eating the apples be conscious of chewing the apples thoroughly. When you feel hungry, simply eat another apple!

As well as eating apples through the day you need to drink filtered warm water. Consuming only cold fruit is not ideal for the digestive system so the warm water is an important part of the regime.

On day 3 eat apples as before, with warm water. You will probably notice that you continue to have bowel movements through the three-day regime. However, on this night before you go to sleep take four tablespoons of olive oil and wash it down with some warm water. As mentioned in Chapter 7, when olive oil is taken it encourages the flow of bile and release of liver toxins that are ready to be released because of the fast.

On day 4 you can gently break your fast. Take some fruit in the morning, at midday have some steamed vegetables, and by the evening you can have some kind of soaked porridge with oats, quinoa or buckwheat, or a watery soup with rice.

This is a surprisingly effective cleanse and ideal if you haven't the time, inclination or constitution to do a more extreme detox.

Vegetable fast

The vegetable fast is common in Ayurvedic retreats. Steamed vegetables are consumed, usually alongside the water from cooked lentils (dhal). It is easier on the body than a fruit-only fast and normally involves between three and six meals each day. Commonly used vegetables are broccoli, carrots and potatoes and slow careful chewing of the food is strongly encouraged. The vegetable fast is very easy to follow and ideal for people who feel the cold. The dhal water is also a highly concentrated source of protein which can make the detoxification process less drastic and enable more fragile people to undertake cleansing.

Lemonade fast

Not quite as radical as water fasting (but almost), the lemonade fast involves a mixture of lemon juice, cayenne pepper, water and maple syrup (these are the same ingredients as in the kidney flush). Originally called the 'Master Cleanse', it was created by Stanley Burroughs in the 1950s. It is very cleansing, especially for the kidneys, but more sustainable for many people, thanks to the maple syrup.

HOW TO DO THE LEMONADE FAST

The mixture contains:

   2 tbsp organic lemon or lime juice

   2 tbsp organic maple syrup

   $1/10$ tsp cayenne pepper

Simply place the ingredients in a 300ml glass and fill with warm water. Then stir until the maple syrup is dissolved.

The recommended dosage is anything between six and twelve glasses throughout the day, although more can be taken if you get hungry. However, given the potentially detrimental effect of the maple syrup and lemon juice on the enamel of the teeth, you may wish to drink the mixture through a straw. At the very least I would recommend swilling your mouth with cold water throughout the day.

Many advocates of this cleanse explain that, to keep the bowel movements regular, it is essential to take either a laxative, such as soaked linseeds (see page 110), or an internal salt wash made from a litre of lukewarm water and two level teaspoons of rock salt. Just stir the salt into the water and drink the entire mixture first thing each morning.

Although I've not recommended this routine to my patients, I know many people who have undertaken this cleanse.

Water fast

This simply involves just drinking water. Most people can manage a day of water fasting, and in many cases it is a beneficial process to go through. Some people enjoy beneficial effects by fasting for one day a week. Water fasting for more than one day should be done under professional supervision.

JUICE FASTING

When fasting, fat gets broken down and soluble toxins such as pesticides, insecticides and petrochemicals that may have been in the body for several years are released into the bloodstream. It is essential to eliminate these from the body as quickly as possible as they are often highly dangerous. For this reason, keeping the elimination channels, such as the bowels and sweat glands, functioning is highly important.

If you are thinking of embarking on a fast for the first time, I would recommend that you start with trying the three-day apple diet, while carefully monitoring your reactions and how you feel.

If you want to embark on a liquid fast then I would usually only recommend a juice fast. Although fasting on water has a good therapeutic history I find for many it can be too drastic. This is especially the case if there are environmental toxins in the body, which is the case for most people. Water doesn't contain antioxidants, enzymes and nutrients, which are essential for the elimination of these toxins. When we take in juices it is much easier to metabolise and excrete these toxins.

Juices are incredibly rich in nutrition. One of my teachers, Richard Schulze, a natural healer from the USA, believes that taking juices is like having a natural blood transfusion. Most of the fibre in produce is removed in the juicing process. This makes it easy to digest and absorb the nutrition. Much less energy is needed by the body to absorb nutrition from a juiced carrot than from eating a whole vegetable. Of course, in an everyday diet, fibre is important, but in a cleanse we want to channel as much of the body processes towards healing as possible. When consuming juice you are resting the digestive system while massively increasing the quality of nutrients. In a single juice you could consume the goodness of two carrots, an inch of cucumber, a beetroot and one stick of celery all at once. Far harder would be to munch your way through the produce with all the fibre that entails.

The nutrition in juice is bio-available, meaning that the body can absorb and utilise the vitamins and minerals it contains. This is not always the case with some synthetic vitamins and minerals as they are not always absorbed. Juices are normally assimilated in a short period of time, usually in about 30 minutes, and thanks to all the enzymes, vitamins and minerals they provide, they improve the whole biochemical environment of the body.

The Gerson Therapy is an alternative cancer treatment developed by Dr Max Gerson in the 1930s (see Gerson and Walker 2001). That, too, involves the intake of freshly prepared juices.

When fasting on juices it is common to experience sporadic hunger pangs during the first few days. This usually passes by the third or fourth day.

Which juices should we use?

The first thing to say about juice fasting is that whatever juice you use, make sure it is extracted from organic produce. The last thing you need is a glass of pesticides in your healing juice. Second, for cleansing purposes, juices from vegetables are generally better than those from fruits.

To get the best health benefits from juices, they need to be freshly prepared each time and consumed within five minutes. This is because the enzyme and nutrient content will oxidise and degrade if the juice is left standing. If you have difficulty preparing the juices this way, you can make two portions, for hourly consumption, and refrigerate until needed. If you're travelling, you can also store the juice in a thermos flask quite safely.

Some juices are more detoxifying than others. Fruit juices contain more sugar than vegetable juices and can create disturbances in blood sugar levels when fasting.

As well as the vegetables mentioned in the box on page 133, lettuce, cucumber, kale and parsley are excellent cleansers when juiced. The greener the juice, the more cleansing and alkalinising it is, but also the stronger tasting it is, so you can vary it as you wish.

You can use lemon, as although it is acidic it has an overall alkaline effect on the body. Ginger is another great addition to a juice. As well as improving the taste and digestion, it is warming, so will help your temperature and circulation.

Although fruit should usually be avoided when doing a juice fast, apples are an exception and can be added to any of the juice recipes and combinations.

Each vegetable has its own particular healing quality. Carrots, for example, are high in beta-carotene, which the body can convert into vitamin A. Beta-carotene is also particularly good at healing skin disorders and the digestive tract. Beetroot, meanwhile, is high in iron and trace elements and improves the quality of blood. So, the wider your variety of juices, the better your intake of nutrients.

EXAMPLES OF JUICE RECIPES

2 carrots

1 small beetroot

1 stick celery

1 small piece ginger

¼ lemon

For an even more powerful cleansing effect, add more greens to the juice. This will both increase the rate of detoxification and intensify alkalinisation – thereby speeding up the elimination of toxins. So, for a slightly stronger mixture, try a recipe with a higher percentage of green vegetables. Use equal parts of:

beetroot

brussels sprouts

carrots

celery

green peppers

spinach

Restoring the acid–alkaline balance

Most people's diet involves the intake of excessively processed foods such as bread, pasta, sweets, dairy and meat products. These foods are essentially acidic in nature, so if the body is a little alkaline then it is generally healthy and resistant to disease.

The pH of the body is a very fine balance. A number of complex processes keep this maintained. Minerals such as magnesium, calcium, sodium and potassium are necessary to keep the system alkaline. We also need a reserve of these minerals in the tissues of the body, without which the body will raid our bones and muscles for calcium and magnesium. This is why excess protein and acidic food can cause some types of osteoporosis – they deplete the calcium store in the bones. Many types of fatigue are related to low levels of magnesium in the body, which can be caused by, or accentuated by, an acidic diet and lifestyle.

How long can you juice fast for?

Most people can manage at least a one-day fast. This means abstaining from food for 24 hours and consuming only liquids. I have set out a sample seven-day cleanse below which involves a five-day juice fast. This is suitable for most people, being cleaning and detoxifying without being too intense. I frequently put patients on ten-day juice fasts over a number of months for various health complaints.

A fasting regime needs to be suitable to your body type and any medical conditions need to taken into account. If you are already thin or underweight, for example, lengthy fasts may be counterproductive. Instead you may need cleansing regimes which work a little bit more slowly, but allow you to maintain a healthy calorie intake. Most people, however, can undertake a one-day fast with no problems.

Who shouldn't fast?

Fasting should not be undertaken by anyone unless under the guidance of suitably qualified practitioner. Fasting is not suitable for people:

- who are pregnant
- who are taking medical drugs
- with diabetes, heart disease, kidney disease or liver disease
- with Parkinson's disease
- who have a history of eating disorders.

What type of juicer do I need?

There are many types of juicer, the most common being the centrifugal juicer. They are the cheapest and easiest available; however, a lot of the nutrition such as vitamins, minerals and enzymes are lost by using them.

The best ones are worm-gear or twin-gear masticator juicers because they keep juices cooler and provide a far higher juice yield than the centrifugal models. The antioxidant and enzyme concentration is also higher – and therefore more effective.

THE SEVEN-DAY INTENSIVE JUICE FAST

The seven-day juice fast involves abstaining from all food, including the vegetables that you may be juicing. Any amount of eating can restart your digestive processes, which would be counterproductive. The aim is to consume four litres of fluid daily. You should never feel really hungry on this fast. If you do…simply drink more.

Fresh vegetable juices will flood your body with health-building enzymes, vitamins, minerals and other essential nutrients.

During the fast avoid using any chemical soaps, shampoo, hairspray, deodorants, make-up or talcum powder. Toothpaste must be fluoride-free. I also recommend avoiding television, especially news programmes, and treating your fast as an opportunity for contemplation and reflection.

YOUR SEVEN-DAY JUICE FAST SHOPPING LIST

1 sack of organic (washed) carrots

1 sack of organic apples

some loose organic beetroot, celery, potatoes, dark
    greens and onions

organic garlic, lemons, virgin olive oil and fresh ginger
    root

1 bag of detox tea (see page 141)

bowel cleanse formula (see page 110)

1 tub of Nutrifood (a vitamin and mineral concentrate,
    which provides additional nutrition and cleanses the
    bloodstream)

500ml flaxseed oil (contains high amounts of omega
    3 and 6, essential fatty acids, and is useful when
    detoxifying and as a daily nutritional supplement.
    Available from most health food shops)

2kg Epsom salts (available very economically in bulk
    from equine supply stores, as it's a remedy for colic
    in horses)

essential oils for your bath

cayenne pepper and filtered water

EQUIPMENT YOU'LL NEED

a juicer

a blender/liquidiser

an empty jam jar

EXAMPLE SEVEN-DAY
INTENSIVE JUICE FAST

Here is an example of a seven-day intensive juice fast. Feel free to modify it to fit your own circumstances and lifestyle. The quantities are approximate and can be varied if necessary.

Day 1
The first day's intake comprises the liver flush (see page 157), salads, mineral broth (see page 140) and freshly made juices.

7.15 am Start your day by drinking 250–400ml of filtered water that is at room temperature, which will help to flush away toxins that have accumulated overnight.

7.30 am Prepare and drink the liver flush. Start simmering the detox tea (see page 141).

7.45 am Drink the detox tea. You can also drink this cleansing tea throughout the day.

8.00 am Shower. Alternate between hot and cold water for a few minutes towards the end of your shower.

9.00 am 400ml fresh vegetable juice (carrot, apple, a little beetroot or celery).

11.00 am Another 400ml juice.

12.00 noon	Lunch on day 1 is mineral broth and a huge salad of sprouted seeds, nuts and steamed vegetables. Make a salad dressing with olive oil, lemon juice, and any herbs and spices you fancy.
2.00 pm	Diluted juice (50% juice, 50% water).
3.00 pm	Diluted juice.
4.00 pm	Diluted juice.
5.00 pm	Diluted juice.
6.00 pm	Diluted juice.
7.00 pm	Diluted juice.
9.00 pm	Hot relaxing bath with essential oils and four cups of Epsom salts.

Days 2 to 6

From days 2 to 6 you will be exclusively juice flushing. This means consuming high quality juices and other fluids such as water, detox tea and mineral broth. No solids are involved in days 2 to 6. Perform an enema at some point during each day.

7.15 am	Upon waking drink 250–400ml of filtered water.
7.30 am	Prepare and drink the liver flush, start simmering the detox tea. (Start preparing mineral broth on days 2, 4 and 6. On days 2 and 4 you should prepare a sufficient amount for two days.)
7.45 am	Drink detox tea.
8.00 am	Shower. Finish by showering your body with alternate hot and cold water for two minutes.
8.30 am	Prepare and drink the bowel cleanse formula (see page 110).
9.00 am	300ml juice.
10.30 am	Bowel cleanse formula.
11.00 am	300ml juice.
12.00 am	300ml juice, blended with two tablespoons of Nutrifood and one tablespoon of flaxseed oil.
12.30 am	Bowel cleanse formula.
2.00 pm	300ml juice.

3.00 pm Mineral broth.
4.00 pm 300ml juice.
4.30 pm Bowel cleanse formula.
5.00 pm 300ml juice.
6.00 pm 300ml juice, blended with two tablespoons of Nutrifood and one tablespoon of flaxseed oil.
6.30 pm Bowel cleanse formula.
7.00 pm Mineral broth or 300ml juice.
8.00 pm Optional detox tea.
9.00 pm Hot relaxing bath with essential oils and four cups of Epsom salts.

Day 7 – breaking the fast

By now, your body will have reached an elevated state of detoxification, so it is very important to break the fast properly. The 'fire of digestion' has to be rekindled, so day 7 involves reintroducing food to the body in a careful, measured fashion.

7.15 am Upon waking, drink 250–400ml of filtered water.
7.30 am Prepare and drink the liver flush. Start simmering the detox tea.
7.45 am Drink detox tea.
8.00 am Shower. Finish by showering your body with alternate hot and cold water for two minutes.
8.30 am Prepare and drink the bowel cleanse formula (see page 110).
9.00 am 400ml juice.
10.30 am Bowel cleanse formula.
11.00 am 400ml juice.
12.00 am 400ml juice, blended with two tablespoons of Nutrifood and one tablespoon of flaxseed oil.
1.00 pm Fresh fruit. Chew this very slowly and mix each mouthful with plenty of saliva to activate the digestive system. Eat until satisfied, not full. You can always eat more later if you're still hungry.

Through the afternoon drink fresh ginger tea, then:

3.00 pm Eat a small vegetable salad.

Evening Eat a plate of steamed vegetables. You can add olive oil, fresh herbs such as torn basil, and some black pepper with a little bit of cayenne pepper.

9.00 pm Hot relaxing bath with essential oils and four cups of Epsom salts.

MINERAL BROTH

A great-tasting part of your cleansing programme is mineral broth. This will stimulate the excretion of inorganic minerals and provide a source of organic minerals.

100g potato peelings

100g carrot peelings and whole chopped beetroots

100g onions and garlic

100g celery and dark greens

2 litres filtered water

cayenne pepper to taste

Place the ingredients in a large pot and simmer on a very low temperature for one to two hours. Strain and drink the broth only and use the vegetables for compost. Mineral broth can be refrigerated and enjoyed the following day.

DETOX TEA

This tea is a special blend of herbs and spices. Digestion stimulating teas are common in ancient systems of medicine. Each herb in the formula is well known for being able to stimulate the digestive process and soothe the stomach as well as being mildly cleansing for the blood, skin, liver and gallbladder. It assists in purifying the bloodstream and the lymphatic system while detoxifying the whole body.

This tea can be drunk at any time and is specifically used with liver cleansing. It contains no caffeine yet is strong tasting to help you get off the tea and coffee habit.

The different herbs in this tea are individually renowned for their therapeutic qualities. Listed below are just two or three of the various qualities that each possesses:

To make your blend of tea blend equal parts by weight of the following ingredients.

Roasted dandelion root (Taraxacum officinale) is considered a common 'garden weed' but has a wealth of health benefits. Rich in vitamins A and C and other minerals, the fresh leaves treat the urinary tract and detoxify the blood. For the purpose of the tea the dried roots are used. The roots reduce inflammation and stimulate the flow of bile.

Burdock root (Arctium lappa) is considered to be one of the best herbal cleansers. Its medicinal properties support the skin and kidney function and alleviate congestion in the lymphatic system. It has a potent anti-inflammatory action, believed to be because of the presence of arctigenin (Zhao, Wang and Liu 2009).

Cinnamon (Cinnamonum zeylanicum) is an aromatic herb commonly used in cooking. It adds flavour to the tea as well as being an excellent digestive stimulant and optimising the production of hydrochloric acid in the stomach. Cinnamon has been shown to have a powerful blood sugar reducing effect. It is thought that the constituent hydroxychalcone found in cinnamon is responsible for its insulin optimising action (Khan *et al.* 2003).

Cardamom seeds (Elettaria cardamomum) are warming and soothing to the digestive tract. They relieve digestive cramping and griping and also have antiseptic qualities.

Liquorice root (Glycyrrhiza glabra) is known as the universal herb. It has a long history in the East, China and Egypt, and was carried by the armies of Alexander the Great as a medicine. It is very soothing and softens the mucous membranes. It is anti-inflammatory, a mild laxative and increases gastric juices. It is a liver protective and is healing to the glandular system, particularly the adrenals.

Fennel seeds (Foeniculum vulgare) are good for delicate stomachs. This is another warming herb that aids digestion, relieving wind and digestive gases.

Juniper berries (Juniperus communis) were used for many illnesses by some of the North American Indian tribes. They aid the digestion, remove waste from the bloodstream and strengthen the brain and the memory. Specific for the kidneys, bladder and urinary passages.

Ginger root (Zingiber officinale) works as a great antispasmodic as well as a stimulant. It helps to reduce the feeling of nausea that some people experience with a liver flush, and is considered to increase circulation to the muscles in Chinese medicine. It reduces the symptoms of aching muscles after exercise (Black *et al.* 2010).

Clove buds (Eugenua caryophyllata) warm the body, increase the circulation and stimulate the organs of excretion as well as disinfecting the liver, kidneys, skin and bronchioles. It has a good flavour and aids the digestion.

Black peppercorns (Piper nigrum) are an excellent digestive stimulant. They are specifically good for drying out 'damp contions', so help the body deal with dysbiosis and yeast overgrowth. The volatile oils have a vermifuge effect, which means they kill parasites and worms.

Orange peel (Citrus sinensis) contains vitamin C, has digestive promoting properties and promotes anti-inflammatory immune processes.

Parsley root (Petroselinum crispum) is a diuretic and its historic uses have been for promoting the breakdown of stones and calcium deposits.

How do I make detox tea?

Add two tablespoons of the dried herbal mixture to 1¼ litres of filtered water. Soak overnight and in the morning simmer for 15 minutes. Drink liberally throughout the day for the duration of the liver flush or juice fast.

WHAT FASTING CAN DO FOR YOU

The long list of conditions that fasting can help to alleviate include the following.

Physical:
- acne
- allergies
- arthritis
- autoimmune diseases
- chronic poisoning
- degenerative disorders

- digestive disorders
- gallstones
- headaches
- hay fever
- high blood pressure
- migraines
- psoriasis
- trauma.

Mental (under supervision):

- depression
- schizophrenia.

Fasting can also help us to deal with our emotions and our spiritual side.

Emotional:

- gives us time and opportunity to deal with emotional issues and to let go of old patterns
- allows us to gain perspective on our feelings.

Spiritual renewal:

- allows us to become aware of our attachments to food and our senses
- enables us to connect with our self and our true spiritual nature
- helps us to realise that we are more than just our physical body.

Many people believe that fasting is the same as starving. It most definitely is *not* the same thing at all. When taking juices, for example, there is plenty of nutrition in the routine, especially when supplemented by superfood powders such as spirulina.

It is interesting to note that some people have endured lengthy spells without food, which is feasible where there is sufficient weight to lose. One obese man fasted – under medical supervision – for over 382 days, consuming just water. He lost 125kg (19 stones) (Stewart *et al.* 1973).

Short fasts can be really beneficial for most people; the emphasis is not on the absence of food, but on providing your body with lots of easily digestible nutrients for a short period of time to promote and encourage cleansing and healing.

For the final word on fasting, let's return to the Essene Gospel of Peace at the Vatican:

> Purify, therefore, the temple that the Lord of the temple may dwell therein and occupy a place that is worthy of him. Renew yourself and fast. For I tell you truly that…plagues may only be cast out by fasting. (Szekely 1981)

Warning: When fasting and cleansing, please be aware that the absorption and therefore potency of medical drugs can alter. Therefore, fasting should never be carried out with out medical supervision. For example, the contraceptive pill might not be effective due to potentially faster bowel transit time. Any type of cleansing should only be undertaken with the personal guidance of a suitably qualified practitioner. If you experience any unusual and/or uncomfortable symptoms during a cleansing regime, you should stop the routine immediately. Symptoms such as dizziness, fatigue, nausea, trembling and rapid heart rate can be signs of electrolyte imbalance and medical advice should be sought immediately. Fasting can be contraindicated for those who have received chemotherapy at any time, as residues of the drugs can be released into the bloodstream and create toxicity. It can also be contraindicated for alcoholics, those who have (or have a history of) eating disorders, diabetics, substance users, those with neurological conditions and pregnant women.

Chapter 7

THE LIVER AND GALLBLADDER

THE LIVER

The liver is sited on the right-hand side of the body beneath the rib cage. It is the heaviest of all internal organs. The liver performs many vital processes – more than 500 functions that we know of, and probably more besides. It enables the body to absorb what it needs to be healthy and to detoxify the rest. The liver:

- stores and assimilates vitamins, minerals and sugars

- metabolises proteins and carbohydrates, enabling the production of energy

- cleans the blood, filtering out bacteria, chemicals and toxins such as pesticides

- removes pharmaceuticals and alcohol from the bloodstream

- produces bile, which among other things enables fat to be broken down

- creates important immune-enhancing substances

- produces important co-factors which allow oestrogen and other hormones to work properly

- keeps the levels of hormones in balance by producing and breaking down oestrogen and testosterone
- produces up to a litre of digestive fluids a day.

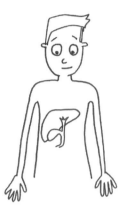

The liver protects us from the onslaught of the modern world. With the toxic effects of man-made chemicals on the increase, we may be ingesting additives or pesticides unwittingly, or being exposed to them from our environment. Most chemicals and toxic substances are fat-soluble, so can reside in the body's fat deposits. The liver itself can also hold toxins because it stores fats such as essential fatty acids and fat-soluble vitamins such as A, D and E.

One way in which the liver detoxifies chemicals is by turning them from a fat-soluble form to the more manageable water-soluble form. This enables us to eliminate these substances through urine, sweat or faeces. The liver has the task of neutralising and transforming pollutants that enter the body. Remarkably, almost all the blood in the body is filtered through the liver every three to four minutes. During this process, the liver deals with any metabolic waste naturally produced by the body and removes other foreign substances such as pharmaceutical drugs, alcohol and caffeine. Some of this waste will be released into the digestive tract via the bile ducts. This is why herbs and cleansers that stimulate bile flow promote detoxification.

What can go wrong?

Most of the patients I see are unaware that the liver is involved in their health issues. Orthodox medicine doesn't tend to identify an under-functioning liver; it is only when the liver is seriously diseased or when liver enzymes are found to be elevated that it is highlighted as a problem. However, there are many stages in between a fully functioning, healthy liver and a liver that is struggling and diseased.

Table 7.1 Stages of liver health

Healthy liver	Sub-optimum	Diseased
Digests fat easily	Headaches	Episodes of jaundice
Good digestion without bloating	Acid reflux from fatty foods	Gallbladder pain
Clear skin	Often feel nauseous	Liver inflammation
Healthy relationship with anger	Irritable, depressed	Cirrhosis
	Skin problems	

Table 7.1 lists some of the signals we receive from an unhealthy liver. Most of us get subtle warnings that something may be wrong. Our bodies are always attempting to communicate with us but we don't always understand its language. Ancient medicine is based on understanding the subtle messages that the body gives us through a combination of signs and symptoms. In Chinese medicine, one way to assess someone's liver is by their tone of voice. Other signs include a green colouring on the face and the shape and colour of the tongue.

In modern medicine, symptoms are often seen as random occurrences that need to be suppressed. We can take paracetamol for a headache, but if the root of that headache is a problem in the liver, the paracetamol will, eventually, make things worse.

Often, symptoms only become severe when the underlying problem is well developed. With hepatitis C, for example, there may be no direct liver symptoms for many years, although an individual may frequently feel tired.

Sometimes it is not clear which symptoms are coming from the liver. Many come from a number of stresses, such as the bowel and lymphatic congestion. That said, I urge almost all of my patients to do a liver cleanse, even if their symptoms do not appear to correlate directly to that organ. Some people notice direct results, such as improved skin condition or, for women, easier periods. Other patients may not notice any change straight away, but will benefit from a reduced toxic load in their bodies later on.

How the liver detoxifies

DETOXIFICATION PATHWAYS

The liver has two main detoxification pathways, Phase I and Phase II:

- *Phase I.* Phase I involves the transformation of a fat-soluble toxin. Through the Cytochrome P450 enzymes, some toxins are made water soluble (like caffeine) and can be excreted by the kidneys. Other toxins are only partly detoxified and can be made more toxic until processed by Phase II.

- *Phase II.* In Phase II the liver enzymes add another substance to the partly broken down toxin if necessary. This is called 'conjugation'. This renders the toxin water soluble so it can then be excreted through the bile and out through the bowel, or through the kidneys.

Both processes have to be working well for detoxification to work effectively. A complicated enzyme process makes all this possible. The most common enzyme in Phase I detoxification is Cytochrome P450. This is our most powerful detoxification enzyme, yet it can be disrupted by xenobiotics such as chemical drugs and pollutants.

Phase II requires a compound called glutathione. This is a tripeptide, a mixture of three amino acids – cysteine, glutamine and glycine – that are synthesised by the body to produce a powerful antioxidant. Glutamine and glycine are normally abundant in the Western diet; however, cysteine, which is needed in large amounts for the creation of glutathione, is frequently deficient. While the body can create cysteine from another amino acid, methionine, most people are short of dietary sources of glutathione. Sulphur is a constituent of cysteine and therefore of glutathione.

Glutathione is present in every cell in the body, with the greatest concentration being in the liver. For various reasons the liver can become depleted of this substance, most commonly when metabolising large amounts of toxins. Other causes of glutathione depletion can be intake of alcohol, bacterial and viral infections and recreational drugs. When this happens, detoxification is compromised.

To maintain the correct level of glutathione and its precursors, it is essential that there is enough sulphur in the diet.

For fully effective detoxification, both phases need to be working. While some toxins can be completely detoxified by either phase alone, others can only be eliminated by a combination of Phase I and Phase II.

A common scenario is where toxins are broken down in Phase I in preparation for Phase II. These broken-down substances, or metabolites, are highly unstable and can, at this stage, be even more toxic than in their original form. The body needs sufficient antioxidants to cope with these toxic metabolites before they go into Phase II. Without enough of the base ingredients such as sulphur and glutathione – and the vitamins and minerals that allow this process to work properly – detoxification becomes slow.

Genetic factors are also involved, with some people better able to detoxify than others. Nevertheless, by reducing our toxic load and maintaining the right ingredients in our diet, we can improve detoxification.

What can stop the liver from functioning properly?

The liver's capacity to repair itself is incredible. With just 25 per cent of its tissue remaining after surgery, it can regenerate itself to its original size within a few months.

Factors affecting the health of the liver include:

- fats
- chemicals and drugs (xenobiotics)
- alcohol
- stress
- infections.

FATS

While some fats are vital for good health and vitality, others, especially fried and heated oils and excess animal fats, are difficult for the liver to process. Worse are artificially created fats such as hydrogenated or trans-fats as their chemical make-up is similar to plastic – which is disastrous for liver function.

Cholesterol is naturally produced in the liver for healthy processes in the body. It is needed to protect the arteries from deterioration from toxins like heavy metals, for example. Unfortunately, excess cholesterol can block arteries and cause heart disease. Meat and dairy contribute to higher cholesterol levels, as do hydrogenated fats. Modern medicine frequently prescribes statins, which shut down some of the liver function in order to reduce cholesterol levels. However, I do not believe that this addresses the underlying causes.

Tests that determine homocysteine levels in the blood are gaining in popularity. Elevated concentrations of this naturally occurring chemical in the blood seem to be a key factor in heart disease and Alzheimer's as homocysteine inflames the arteries. This may be more important than cholesterol in assessing the risk of heart disease and strokes. A deficiency of certain B vitamins and toxic overload are common causes of increased homocysteine.

When people are overweight, fat builds up in the liver. A fatty liver, one of the most common causes of liver disease, creates inflammation and scarring. A healthy weight, therefore, is important to the health of the liver.

CHEMICALS AND DRUGS

Pesticides, insecticides, plastics, pharmaceutical drugs and chemicals such as formaldehyde can seriously hamper healthy liver function. Most chemical drugs include liver damage in their list of possible side-effects, the main offenders being chemotherapy drugs, anti-inflammatories, steroids and painkillers. An overdose of pharmaceutical drugs can cause liver toxicity, while an overdose of paracetamol can destroy the cells in the liver.

Chemicals have an affinity for fat cells and can remain in the body for years. If the toxic burden is significant, the body retains these chemicals unless the elimination channels are working properly. This prevents them from settling in other tissues and creating further damage and is why some people struggle to lose weight. Rapid weight loss can cause some of these toxins to be released, resulting in headaches, insomnia, tiredness and irritability. Moving to a more gradual programme of weight loss, and good bowel cleansing, should prevent these symptoms from being too severe.

ALCOHOL

Alcohol places a huge burden on the liver. When the body breaks alcohol down it first converts it into acetaldehyde, a chemical far more toxic than alcohol and which gives the feeling of a hangover, a common symptom of which is a headache. This has to be metabolised through the liver and the detox pathways before being converted into an easier and more manageable acetic acid. When alcohol levels are high, acetaldehyde leaks into the bloodstream from where it can affect the neurotransmitters in the brain. If the body cannot convert this surplus acetaldehyde into acetic acid then there is a real risk of poisoning. Some people have a genetic weakness which prevents them from transforming acetaldehyde into acetic acid. East Asians and some indigenous peoples are notable examples, with approximately 50 per cent of these populations unable to metabolise alcohol. Their toxic reactions to acetaldehyde – and therefore the effects of drinking alcohol – include nausea, headaches, dizziness and facial flushing.

Liver cirrhosis

Liver cirrhosis occurs when damaged liver cells are replaced by scar tissue instead of new, healthy cells. The most common causes of liver cirrhosis are excessive and prolonged alcohol use and the hepatitis C virus. The majority of people who develop liver damage from hepatitis C are unaware that they have the virus, meaning that serious liver diseases can go unnoticed. Cirrhosis and hepatitis should be managed by a qualified practitioner.

STRESS

When the body experiences stress, anxiety or emotional pressure, it produces chemicals such as adrenalin and cortisol. Excessive levels of these chemicals are broken down in the liver.

INFECTIONS

Our liver helps us to fight infection, both by removing bacteria and viruses out of the blood and by producing macrophages, which destroy bacteria in the gut.

Hepatitis

Medical terms ending with 'itis' mean inflammation. Hepa refers to the liver. Hepatitis therefore means inflammation of the liver. Broadly speaking there are two types – a sudden, acute inflammation and chronic inflammation developing over time. The majority of cases are caused by infection of the hepatitis virus types A, B or C. Less common are viruses that can also cause glandular fever, herpes simplex and yellow fever.

Several symptoms can accompany hepatitis. The most common symptom with acute hepatitis is a yellow tinge to the skin and the sclera, the whites of the eyes. Known as jaundice, this occurs because the liver is unable to process bilirubin, which instead comes out through the skin and in dark coloured urine. With bilirubin no longer excreted through the liver into the bowels, the stools lose their normal brown colour and turn white.

Natural medicine and the liver

Natural medicine uses terms such as a sluggish liver or liver stagnation to describe a liver where the detox pathways are not fully functioning. Symptoms of a sluggish liver can be:

- heaviness beneath the right rib cage
- feeling tired and sluggish in the morning
- bitter/bad taste in the mouth
- eye problems
- difficulty with digesting fatty foods

- irritability

- poor skin – blotchy, spotty, eczema and psoriasis

- headaches and migraines.

When the liver is sluggish and toxic it becomes overheated, giving rise to symptoms such as headaches and inflammations of the skin such as acne and eczema.

Emotional factors and the liver

'It's galling,' 'He is full of bile,' 'I am feeling liverish.' These statements all relate to emotions associated with the liver. In European humeral medicine one of the four temperaments is choleric, which is a reference to bile. William Shakespeare's works are littered with references to 'choler', meaning passion, anger and action.

In Chinese medicine, the term for a sluggish liver translates as Liver Qi Stagnation. Melancholy, depression, moodiness, frustration and anger without an obvious cause, and frequent sighing are common manifestations of Liver Qi Stagnation as the liver is responsible for our ability to have vision and for planning. The Chinese also consider courage to be linked to the size of the gallbladder. In 1984 Margaret Thatcher was congratulated by Deng Xiaoping for having a very large gallbladder.

According to the *Su Wen* (an ancient Chinese medical text):

The liver holds the office of the general of the armed forces. Assessment of circumstances and conception of plans stem from it.

The gallbladder is responsible for what is just and exact. Determination and decision stem from it. (Larre and Rochat de la Vallee 1987)

Hormones and the liver

Premenstrual tension can be related to liver stagnation. Many of the symptoms leading up to the flow of menstrual bleeding can be attributed to the liver, such as tiredness, pain and irritability. Cleansing the liver can have a profoundly harmonising effect on the menstrual cycle. The liver also has a role in regulating and processing testosterone. Excess of this hormone in both men and women is eliminated through the liver. When the liver is stagnant and testosterone is not metabolised properly, irritability, aggression and irregular sexual energy can arise.

Healing the liver

To restore and cleanse the liver we need to:

- increase the flow of bile

- promote detoxification pathways

- protect the liver from any additional damage

- ensure healthy bowel movements for waste to get out.

Promoting the flow of the bile is probably the single most important step in protecting the liver and promoting detoxification. Bile, which is created in the liver, allows waste products such as bilirubin and metabolic waste to be released and environmental toxins in the digestive tract to be eliminated. Bile is stored in the gallbladder and works in a similar way to washing-up liquid, which emulsifies oils when cleaning dishes. Bile enables us to digest fat. If our diet is low in fat, bile stagnates, causing liver detoxification to slow down. I have seen patients who have been on many diets to lose weight end up as 'poor excreters' with weak digestion.

The liver flush

The liver flush stimulates the elimination of waste from the body by increasing the flow of bile and generally improving the detoxification pathways in the liver. It promotes the purification of the blood, improves digestion and can reduce cholesterol levels by improving the overall function of the organ. I have recommended it thousands of times and I have found it very effective in reducing overall toxic burdens.

THE LIVER FLUSH

250ml organic cartoned or bottled apple juice

250ml filtered water

1 whole organic/unwaxed lemon (peeled leaving pith)

1 tbsp organic virgin olive oil

1 clove garlic

½ tsp tumeric powder

a chunk of fresh ginger root about the size of your little toe

Blend all of the ingredients in a liquidiser and drink in the morning. The flush should be made fresh each time and consumed as soon as it is made. Once drunk you need to follow it with a 'detox tea' (a simple version is given on page 141). Alternatively use hot ginger or peppermint tea. Do not eat for at least 30 minutes after the liver flush.

Gradually increase the strength of the liver flush each day by adding one clove of garlic and one tablespoon of olive oil, up to a maximum of four cloves of garlic and four tablespoons of olive oil. Maintain this level until you have finished the flush. Should this make you feel nauseous,

---

reduce the amount of garlic and oil and try increasing in more gradual increments.

The liver flush encourages toxins to be released into the small intestine via the bile duct. For this reason, it is important that the bowels are moving regularly, providing a clear exit from the body. When we are producing and releasing the correct amount of bile, digestion is effective without leaving us feeling tired after eating. The liver flush is also very useful for treating constipation caused by a lack of bile and digestive juices. I recommend that the flush is taken every day for a minimum of one week, but for maximum medicinal benefit it should be taken daily for four weeks.

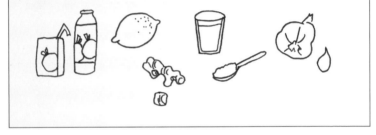

HOW THE LIVER FLUSH WORKS

The liver flush increases the flow of bile from the liver and gallbladder, allowing the body to dump toxins from the liver into the digestive tract, for eventual elimination via the gut. Each ingredient has a favourable influence on the liver function.

- *Apple juice.* This is high in malic acid, which can render toxic metals inert and increase cellular energy. Apple juice also improves the taste of the liver flush.

- *Olive oil.* A sudden quantity of oil through the feedback mechanism in the gut stimulates large amounts of bile to pass into the small intestine.

- *Lemon.* Being sour, lemon activates bile flow and the production of digestive enzymes. It also helps the digestion of the oil and makes the flush palatable.

- *Garlic.* Garlic is antibacterial, antifungal, antiparasitic – and antisocial. If this is a problem, it can be omitted or kept at a low dose in the mixture. Garlic contains over 100 sulphur compounds, so also promotes Phase II of the detoxification pathways. Trials with garlic undertaken over a four-year period showed that plaque deposits on arteries can be reduced by between 5 per cent and 18 per cent (Koscielny *et al.* 1999).

- *Ginger.* This helps to settle the stomach and prevents nausea through the stimulation of digestive juices. Ginger contains gingerol, a chemical that is known to counteract liver toxicity by stimulating bile excretion. It increases the level of the antioxidant enzyme, superoxide dismutase, which protects against oxidative stress.

- *Turmeric.* As mentioned later, turmeric is an incredibly powerful detoxifier and probably the most powerful anti-inflammatory agent in nature.

WHAT TO EXPECT FROM THE LIVER FLUSH

People often say, 'What? Oil and garlic? In the morning?!' It can seem like a strange combination, but is much more tasty than you may first think. Most people are able to take it without any nausea or other digestive disturbances.

A common response after a few weeks of liver flushing is increased energy and vitality. There may also be some healing reactions such as spots for a week or two.

If you have a high level of liver congestion and feel slightly nauseous after the liver flush, reduce the dosage and gradually increase your intake over the course of a few weeks. Drinking detox tea will also help with queasiness. A small number of people get loose stools with the liver flush. Again, reducing the dosage should help your bowels get back to normal.

Case history: Liver flush

Samantha was suffering from extreme tiredness and fatigue and an unexplained, nagging ache between her shoulder blades. Tests carried out by her doctor revealed no evident problem, so Samantha came to my clinic to try a natural approach to her energy problems. While appearing healthy, Samantha told me that in the past she would regularly binge drink. I put her on the liver flush for a month. Six weeks later, Samantha told me that she had more energy and vitality than she had had for years. She woke up in the mornings feeling refreshed and reported that her following menstrual cycle was completely painless.

Herbs and foods for healing the liver

Herbs are excellent for the health of the liver. Across the hedgerows of Britain are plants with an affinity for the liver, with both the sour and bitter tastes promoting the movement of bile. The bitter flavours improve digestion, increase the production of stomach enzymes and normalise the hydrochloric acid levels in the stomach, while sour tastes increase the release of bile.

Many cultures understand the importance of aperitifs, which stimulate gastric juices and the flow of bile prior to a heavy meal. For example, Zwack Unicum, a national drink in Hungary, contains no less than 40 herbs and spices which help the digestion of a diet traditionally high in meat and fat. Another aperitif (or digestif) is the Italian Fernet Branca. Many cultures will use bitter foods, or bitter salads.

Sour foods that help to promote a healthy liver are:

• apples

• apple cider vinegar

• asparagus

- bilberries

- blackberries

- cherries

- greens such as kale and raw sprouted beans

- lemons

- limes

- olives

- plums

- pomegranate

- quinoa.

Some bitter foods to include might be:

- camomile

- celery

- chicory

- dandelion leaves and roots

- lettuce

- radishes

- watercress.

You won't need very much of these foods to have an effect, but place the emphasis on green leafy vegetables.

There are many herbs which can dredge the liver of impurities, protect it from damage and improve its function. Again, most of these have a bitter taste and it is best to take them in the form of a tea or a tincture – as opposed to capsules – as the taste itself is an intrinsic part of its medicinal function.

MILKTHISTLE (*SILYBUM MARIANUM*)

Milkthistle is commonly used in liver treatment as it is a strong liver cell protector. Part of its biochemical mix is the combination of three components called silibinin, silydianin and silychristin. Collectively these are called silymarin. Milkthistle can:

- stimulate the regeneration of liver cells
- protect liver cells from toxins and drugs
- increase liver function
- normalise liver enzymes
- reduce inflammation of the gallbladder
- halt the progression of further disease.

Milkthistle is essential to any liver formula I prescribe. It is particularly indicated for those with liver disease such as hepatitis and cirrhosis and has a favourable effect on the P450 enzyme through its antioxidant properties (Racz *et al.* 1990).

TURMERIC (*CURCUMA LONGA*)

An extraordinary medicine with many healing properties, turmeric is anti-inflammatory, lowers cholesterol levels and has heart and artery protecting effects. It is strongly antibacterial, particularly against *Salmonella*, and can boost insulin. Because of its antioxidant properties, research is currently being conducted in Japan into the anti-cancer actions of turmeric.

DANDELION (*TARAXACUM OFFICINALIS*)

The leaves, roots and stems of dandelion promote the gastric juices. Because of its stimulating effect on the liver and the kidney it has been traditionally used as a spring tonic and for arthritis. Dandelion coffee can be used for the liver and to help reduce inflammation caused by gallbladder stones. Dandelion is also an ingredient in my detox tea.

BARBERRY (*BERBERIS VULGARIS*)

The bark of the barberry root is a strong liver stimulant. It hugely increases the flow of bile and reduces gallbladder inflammation. Many bitter herbs have the capacity to bring down a fever – and barberry is no exception.

FENNEL AND GINGER (*FOENICULUM VULGARE AND ZINGIBER OFFICINALE*)

In a liver formula, fennel and ginger provide the calming and harmonising influence.

HERBAL LIVER FORMULA

A typical formula that I would prescribe for cleansing the liver would be:

  3 parts milkthistle seed (*Silybum marianum*)

  3 parts dandelion root (*Taraxacum officinalis*)

  1 part barberry root bark (*Berberis vulgaris*)

  1 part turmeric root (*Curcuma longa*)

  1 part fennel seed (*Foeniculum vulgare*)

  ½ part ginger root (*Zingiber officinale*)

A basic dosage would be 2.5ml of the tincture three times daily as part of the liver cleansing process and taken for up to a month. This blend can also be made into capsule form. Likewise, one capsule (500mg) of the formula would usually be taken three times daily.

Note: Herbal medicines can be contraindicated if you are taking medical drugs, have a medical condition or are pregnant. Please consult a medical practitioner, pharmacist or qualified herbalist before taking any herbal remedies.

THE GALLBLADDER

Cleansing the gallbladder

Connected to the liver, the gallbladder is responsible for storing bile and maintaining a ready supply for the digestion of fat. Bile can also be an important outlet for toxins processed through the liver. However, dietary factors such as excess dairy, saturated fats, meat and toxicity can cause a build-up of a sand-like substance, which settles in the gallbladder. Over time these small grains can congeal and, together with cholesterol, manifest into gallstones.

Gallstones are an accumulation of bile, cholesterol and salts. Typically, they arise from an imbalance of chemistry in the bile. They then accumulate as a result of toxicity, a diet high in saturated fat or low in essential fats, hormone replacement therapy, inflammation in the gut – such as IBS – and emotional stagnation. It is common to have biliary or gallbladder sludge, usually a mixture of cholesterol, calcium and other toxins. This inhibits digestion and detoxification.

Many people unknowingly have a build-up of stagnant bile and stones in their gallbladder. Only when the stones increase in size or number do they become painful. Pain can be severe and felt in the centre of the upper abdomen, around the shoulders and between the shoulder blades. It can also be confused with heart pain. Furthermore, the gallbladder can get irritated and infect itself with a condition known as cholecystitis.

Women are twice as likely as men to develop gallstones. Nobody knows why, but many experts suspect a hormonal link. Overweight people are more prone to gallstones, as are women taking the contraceptive pill or HRT. It is also more prevalent among people using statins to reduce cholesterol.

The gallbladder flush

This potent cleanse flushes out stagnant bile sediment and stones. If you have a history of gallstones then this can be very helpful; however, if you have been diagnosed with gallstones, make sure you are under the care of a practitioner. While it is possible for a stone to get stuck I have not, in 12 years of practice, ever known this to happen. I would normally advise a patient to complete a full bowel cleanse followed by four weeks of the liver flush before embarking on the gallbladder flush, then finishing up with an enema. So:

Bowel cleanse: 2 weeks

⇓

Liver flush: 4 weeks

⇓

Gallbladder flush: 7 days

⇓

Enema/colonic irrigation

We can all improve our health by clearing sediment out of the gallbladder. The virtues of the gallbladder flush have been known in naturopathy for a number of years, the most recent advocate being the naturopath Andreas Moritz, whose timings I have found to be useful. The version I recommend is outlined in the box below.

THE GALLBLADDER FLUSH

7 litres apple juice

4 tbsp Epsom salts

185ml organic virgin olive oil

enough organic lemons to make 120ml of freshly
  squeezed juice (approx 3 to 4)

800ml water

Days 1 to 6

Drink one litre of packaged apple juice each day. Surprisingly, bottled or cartoned apple juice is best for preparing the liver and gallbladder for this cleanse as, being pasteurised, it seems to soften the stagnant bile in the gallbladder, making this flush more effective. If you can't take apple juice, use lemon juice as an alternative: add the juice of three lemons to a litre of water and drink throughout the day. Be sure to drink plain water afterwards and swill your mouth out so that the lemon juice doesn't damage your tooth enamel.

Day 7

am	Today is a partial fast. As well as a litre of the apple or lemon juice in the morning, you can have fruit for breakfast and snacks up to midday.
2 pm	Nothing is to be eaten from now on – you may only drink water.
6 pm	Mix four tablespoons of Epsom salts with 800ml of water and divide into four servings of 200ml each. Drink your first portion now. It is very bitter so may be more palatable sipped through a straw. Alternatively, down it in one! You can also swill your mouth around with plain water afterwards to get rid of the bitter taste.
8 pm	Drink the second dose of Epsom salts and water mix.
9.45 pm	Ideally, you should wait until you have had a bowel movement before drinking the lemon juice and oil mix. If you haven't, massage your abdomen 36 times clockwise then 24 times anticlockwise to stimulate peristalsis. Press quite deeply and vary the size of the circles.

Squeeze the lemons to extract around 120ml juice, then strain out the seeds and pulp. Pour the juice and 185ml of olive oil into a liquidiser and blend until smooth. You could also use a stick blender.

This is your last chance to visit the toilet before drinking the mixture.

10 pm Stand by your bed and drink the oil and lemon juice mixture as quickly as possible – ideally in one go. If you have to sip it, try to get it down within a few minutes. Now lie down immediately, keeping your head slightly elevated so that you are comfortable and able to keep still for at least 20 minutes. Imagine the mixture cleansing your liver and gallbladder. You may feel twinges as the gallbladder empties the bile and sediment into your digestive tract. After 20 minutes feel free to move around and visit the toilet if necessary. If possible, rest and sleep for the night.

Day 8

6 am Drink the third dose of the Epsom salts and a further cup of warm water. Go back to sleep if you need to.

8 am Drink the final dose of Epsom salts and another cup of plain water.

9 am Drink some freshly juiced apples or bottled apple juice as an alternative.

10 am Have a fruit breakfast and some peppermint or ginger tea. Most people are a bit dehydrated at this stage, so sip water throughout the day. Eat normally from lunchtime onwards.

11 am If possible take a coffee enema (see page 117) or arrange for a colonic that includes a coffee implant. This will dilate the bile ducts and further aid the release of sediment.

WHAT TO EXPECT FROM THE GALLBLADDER FLUSH

Most people pass a number of green coloured stones in their bowel movements during the gallbladder flush. The brightly coloured green ones are generally stagnant bile and congealed olive oil. It is also common to pass grains of bile sand, which look like tiny crystalline bits. These are the precursors to gallstones. You may pass foam and froth in with your bowel movements as well as substantial amounts of bile water. This has been coined the 'Niagara Falls' effect by some of my patients! Actual gallstones are recognisable by their colour; some are dark such as black, brown or very dark green, while others are yellow or white, depending on the biochemical make-up of each stone. After drinking the gallbladder flush the numbers will vary from five or ten to as many as 500 in various colours, shapes and sizes. If you want to know exactly what you have passed, place a sieve over the toilet seat to catch any sediment released from the body.

WHO SHOULDN'T TAKE THE LIVER FLUSH OR GALLBLADDER FLUSH?

Warning: Both the liver flush and gallbladder flush have been carried out successfully by thousands of people. Nevertheless, with the amount of oil involved, the process of liver or gallbladder flushing can result in the gallbladder contracting. Theoretically, a gallstone could become trapped in the bile duct, which could lead to a life-threatening medical emergency such as pancreatitis. It is possible to have gallstones and not have any symptoms but still be 'at risk'. Before conducting gallbladder cleanses it is recommended that you consult a medical doctor who may decide to recommend a suitable scan to ascertain whether or not it is safe to undertake the cleanse.

Pregnant women or anyone with colitis or inflammatory bowel disease should not take the liver or gallbladder flush. Epsom salts are not to be taken if you have kidney disease or a history of renal insufficiency.

These cleanses should only be carried out under suitable medical supervision.

Case history: Gallstones

Rodney had been diagnosed with gallstones and would get abdominal pain from these at least two or three times a week. If he ate a meal high in oil or fat he might feel nauseous to the point of vomiting. He was scheduled to have his gallbladder removed in six months. One of Rodney's friends had had a similar operation but had suffered from IBS ever since. Understandably, Rodney was seeking alternatives to the operation and came to see me.

He started off with a bowel cleanse and the liver flush for one month, along with a strict diet of no dairy and no heated oils. Although he found it difficult he persevered and by the end of the month his symptoms had reduced. He then took the gallbladder flush and released around 600 stones of various sizes. All his abdominal pain disappeared and Rodney felt a dramatic improvement in his sense of wellbeing. A month later he repeated the gallbladder flush and released a further 200–300 stones.

Now free of symptoms, Rodney continued to avoid dairy products but was able to tolerate olive oil and digest fats. After six months a scan revealed that, while some stones were still present, Rodney's gallbladder was now a normal size. I predict that it may take a further six to twelve months for the existing stones to break down. In the meantime, however, Rodney is symptom-free, his digestion is normal and he has chosen to avoid surgery.

QUESTIONS AND ANSWERS

I have been diagnosed with hepatitis C. Can a natural approach help?

The medical approach for hepatitis C is usually interferon, a powerful drug which is effective in 40 per cent of cases but can have massive side-effects. Usually promoting the liver function as well as supporting all the other detox organs works well. I have had cases where interferon has not worked and natural medicine has resolved the virus. I have also had cases where the natural approach hasn't been fully effective. Some patients may decide to use interferon as well as natural methods to support the liver. This will require a team effort involving both the medical and alternative practitioners. Either way, recreational drugs and alcohol should be stopped forever and the viral load monitored regularly so you know where you are with the disease.

There is controversy over liver biopsies. Some feel that biopsies may cause scarring, thereby further compromising the organ. I have seen the viral count come down dramatically with herbs and cleansing, only to shoot back up when a patient drinks coffee and alcohol. A teacher of mine, Christopher Hobbs, has successfully treated many people with hepatitis C where pharmaceutical drugs haven't worked. Christopher recommends drinking plenty of lemon balm tea for its antiviral qualities. Milkthistle and shiitake mushrooms, taken daily, will also reduce the viral count. There are other herbs which can be taken but will need to be prescribed by a herbalist.

Clinical experience has shown that cannabis has to be completely avoided in order to clear the virus from the system, whichever treatment process someone chooses to follow.

I have been diagnosed with gallstones… Can I take the liver flush?

In this situation you must seek the guidance of an experienced practitioner. I have had many, many patients who averted surgery by taking the liver flush. I think that the gallbladder should be kept intact wherever possible. There are rare occasions where chronic sepsis, gangrene or other diseases in the gallbladder have gone past the point of no return, but most patients live a pain-free life with the liver flush.

Will the gallbladder flush hurt?

No. There may be occasional discomfort but there shouldn't be any pain. With the gallbladder flush, the Epsom salts have a dilating and laxative effect, encouraging the bile and waste to be carried out of the body through the bowel movements.

Can I cleanse the liver if I have had my gallbladder removed?

Yes. In fact, liver flushing is especially important if you no longer have a gallbladder. Liver support should be a lifelong consideration now.

I have gallstones and the tiniest bit of oil makes me feel ill. What can I do?

If you are sensitive to oil, take lecithin granules. A single tablespoon, three times a day in some juice will help you metabolise fats. Then start to introduce a little bit of raw olive oil in a modified liver flush. One teaspoon in the flush is enough to get started. To get the bile flowing take bitter herbs and foods. Gradually you will be able to do the liver flush and digest fats again.

I am healthy and want to stay that way. How often should I do the cleanse?

The liver flush should be done at least once a year, ideally in spring. The same goes for the gallbladder flush.

Chapter 8

BLOOD AND THE LYMPHATIC SYSTEM

Blood is liquid life force. It carries oxygen from the lungs to all the different cells in the body, delivering vitamins, minerals, protein and nutrition from the food broken down in the digestive organs. Each cell needs nutrition and produces its own metabolic waste, which has to be excreted from the body for everything to work properly. Blood transports all the good stuff to where it's needed and removes the bad stuff.

Blood is pumped around the body through the arteries, which form a network of capillaries. As these channels get smaller there is space only for the blood plasma – the fluid in the blood. Red blood cells get left behind and this fluid then passes through the membrane of the capillaries. This substance is called interstitial fluid, or tissue fluid. This tissue fluid bathes all of the tissue cells, transferring nutrients while removing waste. The lymphatic system then sucks up the waste in the tissue fluid and classes it as lymph. The lymph contains white blood cells, such as lymphocytes, macrophages and antibodies, which protect the body from infection. Lymph is filtered through the lymph nodes, collecting in the lymphatic duct, which then enters the bloodstream.

Haematology, the study of blood, is of course a huge area of medical study. For the purpose of this book, I shall focus on cleansing and building the blood.

Blood cleansing becomes necessary when we get toxic. Our blood can get congested and thick. Evidence of this is usually high cholesterol, circulatory disorders and heart problems and other conditions. People with autoimmune diseases, chronic fatigue and Gulf War Syndrome (GWS) often have a build-up of poisons in the bloodstream.

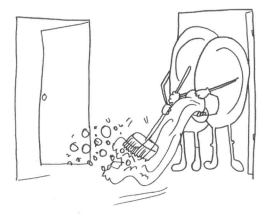

In Chinese medicine, blood stagnation is where the blood does not flow properly within an organ or region of the body. Typical manifestations are varicose veins, menstrual problems and pain. Normally blood stagnation can be seen in a purple colouring of the tongue and nails.

It is said in Chinese medicine that the quality of the blood shows itself in the hair and nails. This makes sense, as anaemic women often get thinning hair and split nails. Blood quality is intimately connected with our emotions and spirit: with sufficient nutrients in our bloodstream, toxins are being processed properly and our mood is more likely to be stable.

Most blood toxicity is a result of poor detoxification of the liver and kidneys and lymphatic burden. The lymphatic system and the blood are intimately connected in a symbiotic relationship.

THE LYMPHATIC SYSTEM

The lymphatic system is essentially the drainage network of the body. Almost all of the cells in the body are surrounded by lymphatic fluid. This receives and filters the waste products from the cells, sending some of the toxins back into the bloodstream to be cleaned by the kidney and liver. Other toxins, especially bacteria and viruses, get filtered through the lymph nodes.

Lymph fluid isn't pumped around the body in the same way as the blood. It relies on the movement of the muscles and limbs for it to flow efficiently through a one-way valve system. Deep diaphragmatic breathing is essential for optimal lymph flow around the body. Lymphatic glands are located all around the body, but the major ones are around the neck, the armpits, the digestive tract, the groin and the knees.

LYMPHATIC CONGESTION

If the lymphatic system gets sluggish, the drainage system slows down. This can result in stagnant lymph and, as a consequence, swelling of the lymphatic glands. Tonsillitis, appendicitis and problems with adenoids can be early signs of lymphatic congestion. The tonsils, appendix and adenoids are all part of the lymphatic system and can be overburdened when the system slows down.

Fortunately, the removal of the tonsils is not as common a practice as it once was. Removing an important line of immune defence shouldn't be undertaken lightly. Usually avoiding dairy and cleaning up the body does wonders for children and adults frequently affected by tonsillitis. I have found that those patients who have had their tonsils removed as children are much more likely to have thyroid imbalances when they get older. The reasons for this are not clear. Perhaps it could be the result of some unseen damage occurring locally during a tonsillectomy.

In cases of glandular fever, where the immune system is attempting to kill the virus, there is often swelling of the lymphatic glands. When there is swelling this is usually a sign that the immune system is mobilising its defences to clear bacteria or viruses. However, it is important that any swelling on the body should always be investigated thoroughly. More than 300 medical conditions can cause swelling of the lymph glands and the cause should be properly identified before starting any treatment.

Signs of lymphatic congestion include:

- appendicitis

- cancer

- cellulite

- chronic fatigue/myalgic encephalopathy (ME)

- fibromyalgia

- frequent bacterial and viral infections

- lumpy breasts

- prostate problems

- skin problems

- swollen lymphatic glands

- tonsillitis.

Causes of lymphatic congestion include:

- alcohol

- constriction, such as with an underwired bra

- diet high in fat, meat, dairy, sugar and refined carbohydrates

- environmental toxins

- infections such as Epstein Barr, mononucleosis, and long-standing infections in the teeth

- lack of exercise and movement

- surgery

- trauma, such as an accident.

Lymphatic congestion can create several conditions. Often with prostate problems in men, there is stagnation in the lymphatic nodes in the groin, the main exit point of cellular toxins from this area. If this congestion continues for long periods of time, the prostate will become overwhelmed with metabolic waste, potentially leading to prostate inflammation and cancer.

The lymphatic glands in the armpits are the main channels where metabolic waste is released from the breast tissues. This means it is important to avoid aluminium and chemicals in deodorants, which could burden the lymph. If body odour is an issue, bowel cleansing and regular skin brushing usually helps.

Some practitioners believe that the rise of breast cancer is, in some part, due to deodorants and underwired bras, which can impair the lymph flow making breast lumps more likely.

To help keep a clean lymphatic system, be very careful what you put on your skin. A herbal teacher once told me she would only put on her skin what she was willing to eat. Products on our skin will get absorbed into our bloodstream. Indeed, many drugs, such as HRT or nicotine patches, are administered this way.

CLEANING THE LYMPHATIC SYSTEM AND THE BLOOD

A free-flowing lymphatic system means a good immune response, less likelihood of falling ill and abundant energy. Good ways to achieve this are:

- exercise and deep breathing

- diet

- skin brushing

- hydrotherapy and saunas

- herbal lymph and blood cleansers

- detox baths

- castor oil packs.

Exercise and deep breathing

Regular exercise is essential to get the lymph moving. Exercise promotes detoxification in the body more than anything else. Activity that results in deep breathing and sweating is not just good for your heart – it also purifies the bloodstream. I have known patients who work with toxic substances or who have atrocious diets, yet remain healthy because they exercise regularly and sweat often. Sweating is particularly good for releasing heavy metals such as mercury. Sweat, which contains urea, lactic acid and other toxins, is very similar to urine in its composition. In naturopathic medicine the skin is classed as the third kidney for its ability to excrete waste from the blood.

Rebounding, using mini-trampolines, which are easily available and cheap, is fantastic exercise and almost anyone can take part. The gravitational force stimulates all the muscles as well as lymphatic flow. It also strengthens your tendons and is a key method of re-mineralising bones.

For many in the Western world, the word exercise summons up visions of daily workouts on the treadmill at the gym. Certainly cardiovascular exercise is important, but it is not the only way to facilitate deep breathing. When we look at ancient cultures that understand the science of longevity, we see a different story. In Ayurveda, the original medical system of India, stretching (yoga) and breathing (pranayama) play a huge part in maintaining health, while in China the effects of tai chi are clear. Every morning, elderly people are in the parks, exercising for a long and healthy life.

Everyone's constitution is different, which means our exercise routines should be different too. Very few of us can go wrong with stretching and walking every day, and swimming is a fantastic exercise for the lymphatic system which doesn't put harmful strain on the joints. Exercising for about 30 minutes three times a week is the minimum most of us need to ensure normal bodily function.

I have treated professional athletes who are technically fit but not healthy. This may be because they place too much emphasis on protein or that they are not achieving the right balance between exercise and relaxation. The most powerful combination, of course, is good exercise, a great diet and quality relaxation.

Diet

A diet rich in fresh vegetables and essential fatty acids is important. Filtered water and the juices of fresh vegetables and fruit should be taken liberally as they provide a wide range of health benefits. Fresh juices such as beetroot and carrot, for example, will clean the blood and increase important nutrients such as iron. Garlic and onions, meanwhile, can promote lymph cleansing.

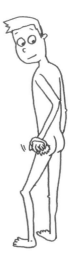

Skin brushing

Skin brushing improves circulation. It can also do wonders for the look of your skin and make you feel refreshed and energised. The benefits to lymphatic flow mean that skin brushing can also reduce cellulite and increase muscle tone, while removing dead skin cells and opening the pores. Because acupuncture meridians flow on the surface and inside the body, skin brushing stimulates the flow of qi and energy through the network of these subtle energy channels. The results are heightened immunity, improved organ function and increased vitality.

How to skin brush

Choose a skin brush made from natural fibres. Synthetic fibres will create an unhealthy static charge. I recommend brushes made from cactus fibre which are available from bodycare shops. They are firm to start with but will soften over time. As skin brushing helps to kick-start the metabolism, it is best done in the morning – it may keep you awake if you do it in the evening.

Directions

Do the skin brush before you shower or wash in the morning. Your skin needs to be dry. Allow between five and ten minutes.

Brush towards the heart. Start at the soles of your feet to activate the reflexology points. From the upper part of the foot, make strokes from the toes toward your ankles.

Brush the skin of each leg vigorously, with the emphasis on the lymphatic glands around your ankles, the back of the knees and your groin. These areas need at least five or six strokes.

Brush up the legs, the thighs and the buttocks, avoiding the genital area. Approach the abdomen with circular clockwise movements. Circle the abdomen three or four times to begin with, then gradually build this up to 12 times over the next few days.

Brush both sides of your hands and work up the inside and the outside of both arms. Make long strokes towards your heart, paying special attention to the inside of the elbows and the armpits. A good skin brush will be too scratchy for your face, but work gently on the sides and back of your neck with downward strokes. Work on your chest but avoid the nipples. Brush as much of your upper back and shoulders as you can reach.

Avoid brushing delicate or irritated skin, varicose veins and any areas affected by eczema of psoriasis.

Follow the skin brush with hot and cold showers for maximum benefit.

Brush every day for a few months, then reduce the frequency to three to four times weekly. This will ensure that your brushing remains effective without your body becoming too accustomed to it.

Make sure nobody else uses your skin brush and wash it regularly with warm water and essential oils – tea tree will keep it clean and bacteria-free. Dry the brush thoroughly to prevent mould growth.

Hydrotherapy and saunas

Greatly underused, hydrotherapy is an ancient medicinal technique which uses water internally and externally. Hydrotherapy can be immensely healing. When the body is exposed to heat, muscles relax and become engorged with blood. Cold then contracts the muscles causing the blood to go deeper into the body. When hot and cold are alternated, a flushing of the body tissues occurs. This combats inflammation, improves circulation and lymph flow and benefits the skin. Some natural spa waters are full of medicinal properties such as sulphur.

Hot and cold therapy is used for healing all over the world and is especially popular across Europe. I have seen some excellent spas in Germany and, most notably, in Budapest in Hungary.

Just one hour in a spa every day for a few months helped one of my patients resolve a seemingly incurable blood disorder.

HOME HYDROTHERAPY

Take a hot shower, then a cold shower. Alternate from hot water to cold, being as extreme as you can with temperatures. When showering, move the water over your skin with the showerhead, in the same directions described for the skin brushing. The more often you alternate the temperature of the water, the greater the benefits for blood circulation, lymph flow and the elimination of toxins. It can also dramatically accelerate injury-healing processes. Most people find a minute at each temperature works well. You may need to build up to the intensity of having the water really cold. Always finish with cold water, letting it run down the back of the neck and along the spine. Scream if you have to! And, if you give yourself a skin brush beforehand, you'll reap even more benefits.

SAUNAS

Saunas create dry heat. They are great for stimulating sweat and releasing impurities. At the beginning of your detox programme start slowly with saunas, spending a few minutes in the heat before having a cold shower. Again, alternating the heat of the sauna with a cold shower will maximise the benefits. Gradually extend the time you spend in a sauna by small increments over a number of sessions. To really increase the amount you sweat, drink hot herbal tea such as peppermint, ginger or the detox tea before taking a sauna.

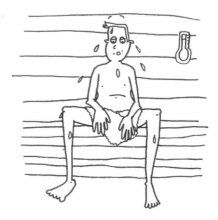

FAR INFRA-RED SAUNAS

More and more is being learned about the detoxifying properties of far infra-red saunas. These provide the same benefits as a regular sauna but at a lower temperature, so are ideal for people who have been advised to avoid regular saunas or intense heat. Infra-red saunas can help mobilise dangerous substances such as organophosphates and petrochemicals and assist their release from the body. Using an infra-red sauna is possibly the most effective way to stimulate the detoxification of man-made chemicals lodged in the body. By measuring the blood before and after infra-red sauna usage, I have seen all kinds of toxins eliminated, such as organophosphates, PCBs, even hair dye that is stored deep within the body's organs. Using infra-red saunas is vital for removing phthalates and bisophenol A.

Sauna detoxification regime

First you need to obtain a far infra-red sauna. Fortunately they are now relatively inexpensive, especially if you obtain a collapsible tent version. Currently they cost about £200.

To eliminate deep-seated toxins, take a sauna for ten minutes every day. Usually it will take at least a month, although with some patients it can take at least six months, for the excretion of these substances. It is important that after the sauna you ingest a teaspoon of bentonite clay and/or activated charcoal.

SWEAT LODGES

A North American Indian tradition, the sweat lodge is conducted according to specific rituals and allows you to sweat emotional and physical toxins from the body. I have attended numerous sweat lodges, all varying in intensity, yet all producing valuable and sometimes profound experiences.

A sweat lodge takes place in a specially constructed dome shaped 'lodge' made from canvas and branches. Hot rocks are placed in the middle and participants sit around them in darkness to create a womb-like environment. The process involves a sequence of rounds: a few minutes of sitting in the warm darkness are alternated with short periods where the entrance is opened to allow fresh air and light to enter before the process starts again.

Herbal lymph and blood cleansers

To clean the blood we need to stimulate all of the body's natural cleansing mechanisms. Fasting is one of the best ways to clean the bloodstream. Herbs that cleanse the blood are called 'alteratives'. Examples are:

- *Cleavers.* A common 'weed' which grows in hedgerows and gardens. When I was at school, we used to throw it at each other, illustrating its common name, 'sticky willy'. It reduces swelling in the lymphatic system and helps to cleanse the blood while stimulating the kidneys.

- *Red clover.* Commonly found in the British countryside, red clover is one of the key ingredients of the famous Hoxsey cancer formula. It is also a blood thinner and has strong antioxidant components.

- *Yellow dock.* Related to common dock, this variety has blood-cleansing properties, stimulates bile flow and increases the absorption of iron.

- *Dandelion.* A powerful diuretic and stimulant for the liver, dandelion contains an assortment of vitamins and minerals.

- *Burdock.* A specific for the blood, though also traditionally used for cleansing the skin, burdock can used internally for eczema, dry skin and psoriasis.

HERBAL LYMPHATIC FORMULA

Here is my blood and lymph cleansing formula:

3 parts dandelion root (*Taraxacum officinalis*)

3 parts burdock root (*Arctium lappa*)

2 parts cleavers (*Gallium aparine*)

2 parts red clover (*Trifolium pratense*)

1 part yellow dock root (*Rumex crispus*)

Each of these herbs is available in a liquid alcohol extract called a 'tincture'. The formula should be made up by blending the specified amounts of the liquid herbal tinctures. Take a basic dosage of 2.5ml to 5ml three times daily for one month while on a lymphatic clean-up.

Detox baths

A detox bath helps to stimulate the skin and lymphatic system and increase magnesium in the body. Start with a five-minute skin brush while the bath is filling with hot water. When the bath is ready, add one cup of cider vinegar and 500g of Epsom salts. Now stand in the bath and rub yourself with a mixture of

100g of Epsom salts and a tablespoon of almond oil. Use brisk circular movements, allowing the mixture to fall into the bath. This again stimulates the skin and the removal of dead skin cells.

Soak in the bath for about 20 minutes and during that time drink a few cups of peppermint or ginger tea. These will make you sweat, so are excellent for getting rid of a cold or flu if you catch it quickly enough. The Epsom salts can promote the release of toxins through the skin and relieve muscle aches and pains. The cider vinegar helps to restore the acid–alkaline balance of your skin, which in turn speeds up the release of metabolic waste.

As mentioned in the section on magnesium, Epsom salt baths help to restock your levels of magnesium (see page 61).

Epsom salts contain a certain type of sulphur which is difficult to find in most foods but can be absorbed through the skin in a detox bath. This is important for many biochemical functions of the body, such as:

- creating digestive enzymes

- maintaining the healthy integrity of the gut wall

- detoxifying environmental pollutants.

(Waring n.d.)

I recommend a detox bath once a week while on a cleansing programme.

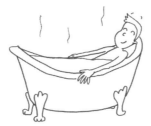

Castor oil packs

Castor oil packs help to clear congestion and stagnation, especially in the lymphatic system, by drawing toxins out of the body through the skin. In naturopathic medicine they are used to reduce pain and inflammation. The American, Edgar Cayce, promoted their healing qualities and recommended them to thousands of people in the 1930s.

Most people are familiar with the use of castor oil for constipation – when taken internally the laxative effect can be dramatic. For detoxification purposes, however, castor oil is applied externally on the skin.

The famous herbalist, Dr Christopher, said that castor oil packs 'get rid of hardened mucous in the body, which may appear as cysts, tumours or polyps' (Christopher 1976). I have used them to help shrink ovarian cysts and fibroids and to reduce pain and inflammation with several patients.

GYNAECOLOGICAL PROBLEMS

Many gynaecological problems are the result of stagnation, constipation and poor blood flow. Known as blood stagnation in Chinese medicine, this can include conditions such as pelvic inflammatory disease, ovarian cysts, fibroids, endometriosis, menstrual irregularity, clotting and some types of sub-fertility. Often the lower abdomen area can feel cold to the touch and will seek relief in a hot water bottle. Keep the lower back warm and apply castor oil packs regularly. This will help to increase the blood flow to the area and speed up healing. I have also known this process relieve the pain of endometriosis.

BOWEL DISORDERS

As castor oil packs can improve lymph flow around the bowel they can also be useful in cases of chronic constipation, particularly for people who have relied on laxatives for a long time. Taken with other measures they can gradually increase the natural tone of the bowel and help in cases of irritable bowel syndrome (IBS) and inflammatory bowel diseases such as colitis and diverticulitis.

Making a castor oil pack

To make a castor oil pack you will need:

> 5–6 tbsp good quality, cold pressed castor oil (see the Resources section)
>
> soft flannel made of cotton or wool (not dyed or bleached)
>
> hot water bottle
>
> small saucepan

Gently heat the castor oil in a pan (not aluminium) to a temperature which is not too hot to touch. Soak the flannel in the castor oil and place on your abdomen. Cover with a towel and place a hot water bottle on top. Now, simply lie down for 45 minutes to an hour. Playing soothing music or just enjoying the silence can enhance relaxation. Focus your mind on the healing process that is now taking place. After an hour, some people then go to sleep and wash the oil off in the morning, while others prefer to clean it off straight away. Either way is fine, but to ensure the oil and the toxins are fully removed from the skin, add two-and-a-half teaspoons of baking soda to a litre of warm water and wash the area where the pack has been with this mixture. Clean again with ordinary soap if necessary.

You (and only you) can use the flannel for up to 30 applications. Store the flannel in a container in the fridge between applications to prevent the oil from becoming rancid.

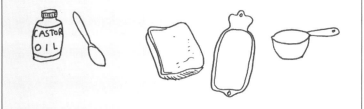

SCARS AND ADHESIONS

Once a wound has healed people can get a residue of scar pain. This can be reduced with regular applications of castor oil packs on the scar and surrounding area. I have seen this work for a soldier who suffered nagging pains from an old bullet wound, especially in the winter months.

NERVOUS SYSTEM

Castor oil packs can also relax the nervous system. In Chinese medicine there is an important acupuncture point below the belly button called the Dan Tien, which is associated with groundedness. Castor oil packs on the abdomen help the body feel centred and have helped in cases of depression, exhaustion and epilepsy.

DETOXIFICATION

Castor oil packs help to clear the lymphatic system and can be used as part of an overall detox programme. As they also enhance the whole immune response, they are useful for people with viral conditions such as glandular fever.

Case history: Fibrocystic breast disease

Tina came to see me with a condition called fibrocystic breast disease. She had numerous lumps in her breasts, which frequent medical tests always showed to be benign (non-cancerous). Tina had had this condition since coming off the contraceptive pill five years earlier. I started by changing her diet, eliminating wheat and dairy and restricting sugar. We then began the process of regular exercise, skin brushing and the liver flush. After one month of the liver flush, Tina noticed a reduction in the size of the lumps. Then, after she had rubbed castor oil regularly into her breasts for around three months, the lumps disappeared completely. Tina now notices that keeping active keeps the lumps at bay, while in periods of inactivity they may reappear.

Case history: Ovarian cyst

Linda was diagnosed with an ovarian cyst, a solid mass 7cm in diameter. She wanted to tackle this naturally as the alternative was to have her ovaries removed. She began a cleansing routine, which involved clearing Candida and drinking ten vegetable juices each day.

She applied castor oil packs three times a week and had localised hot and cold showers on the region of her ovaries. While applying the castor oil packs she would think consciously about ideas and emotions that would arise, as part of the healing process. After six months on this intensive programme no cysts were visible on any scans and Linda's ovaries looked perfectly healthy.

A FREQUENTLY ASKED QUESTION

My child keeps getting bouts of tonsillitis and I don't want to keep giving him antibiotics. What can I do?

A common factor in frequent occurrences of tonsillitis is food intolerance, the usual suspects being dairy and, to a lesser degree, wheat. These can trigger immune responses with a resulting congestion of the lymphatic system. Reduce sugar in the diet and make sure your child gets enough vitamin C. During tonsillitis, drinking pineapple juice and gargling with fresh lemon juice and water can reduce pain and inflammation. Herbal tinctures of echinacea and myrrh will also help. Ingesting three to six fresh cloves of garlic will clear tonsillitis in many cases. Mash some of these into an avocado and chop the rest into little pieces – then swallow them.

Chapter 9

THE KIDNEYS

The kidneys are located at the back of your abdomen on either side of your spine. They are approximately four to five inches (10–12cm) long and around two inches (5cm) wide. They are protected by the ribcage at the back. The kidneys:

- filter metabolic waste such as urea from the blood

- maintain the balance of electrolytes such as sodium and potassium in the blood

- produce the hormone erythropoietin, which stimulates the production of red blood cells in the bone marrow

- manufacture rennin, which helps to regulate blood pressure

- generate calcitriol, which is involved in calcium absorption and utilisation.

The kidneys, like all detoxification organs, are multifunctional. They receive blood via the renal artery and process it through millions of filters called nephrons. The kidneys filter approximately 150 litres of blood every day. This means all the blood in your body goes through the kidneys every 45 minutes. Here, unwanted substances, such as metabolic waste, excess fluid, minerals and salts are removed from

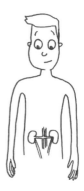

the blood and sent to the bladder for disposal. The kidneys also regulate the acid and alkaline levels in the blood by regulating the pH. A further function is to produce hormones that enable the bone marrow to produce red blood cells, regulate blood pressure and ensure the correct calcium balance in the body.

The kidneys remove huge quantities of substances from our blood. Made up of millions of filters, they can continue to perform even when partially damaged. In fact, most people can easily survive with a single kidney or with each kidney functioning at just 50 per cent of its potential. For the kidneys to function properly the body needs about two litres of fluid a day.

The waste liquid that is filtered by the kidneys is transferred to the bladder through a connection called the ureter, and becomes urine. The bladder, which is like a balloon, then changes size to accommodate the urine. As the bladder fills and approaches capacity, it begins to contract. This is when we feel the need to urinate. We eliminate 1–1½ litres of urine every day.

The kidneys extract toxins that have gone through Phase II detoxification pathways from the blood. However, being designed only to deal with metabolic waste, they are vulnerable to chemicals and heavy metals such as mercury. I have worked with many car mechanics with bad backs which are caused only in part by heavy lifting. A weakness in their kidneys is also a regular feature of their symptoms. Pain can also result from the chemicals, degreasers and petroleum that they are exposed to as these toxins seem to have an affinity to kidney tissue. Kidney cleansing has relieved much of this pain as these chemicals are flushed out. I have also treated several people who work with stained glass and consequently have a build-up of lead in their bodies. Frequently, the kidneys take the brunt of this.

KIDNEY STONES

Kidney stones are a build-up of calcification in the kidney. Not only do they cause great pain, they affect the function of the organ as well, possibly compromising their ability to balance the fluids in the body.

KIDNEY FAILURE

Kidney failure is serious and can result in the need for dialysis, where a machine performs the function of the kidneys. A kidney transplant may be the only alternative to a life on dialysis. Once damaged, kidney nephrons do not regenerate. However, the deterioration of kidney function can be slowed down or even halted with natural treatment. David Winston, a US herbalist, once told me how he had been using stinging nettle seed tincture as the basis for a natural treatment for kidney problems with good results. It is not clear yet how the biochemistry of nettle seeds supports the kidneys but I have also used this tincture with clinical success. Slowing down the rate of deterioration is potentially life-saving for anyone waiting for a kidney transplant.

URINARY TRACT INFECTIONS

Infections in the urinary tract affect women more than men. This is because the woman's urethra, the connection between the bladder and the outside of the body, is shorter than the man's.

A urinary tract infection occurs when bacteria enter the urinary tract and create inflammation. Many women also suffer from occasional cystitis, although many patients can have a low-grade infection for years. The continual prescription of antibiotics for low grade isn't uncommon, but it does give rise to yeast overgrowth. Some people experience symptoms of cystitis continually but reveal no bacterial infection when their urine is tested. Generally the infection is fungal, and cannot usually be detected in routine urine tests. This is especially common in patients with blood sugar imbalance or diabetes. A Candida detox often works wonders with those suffering from longstanding chronic urinary tract infections.

Herbs are excellent for clearing cystitis. I have seen cases of herbs working in a matter of days where antibiotics have had no effect whatsoever. Remember, however, that any infection of the urinary tract can lead to a kidney infection. This can be very serious and, though herbs often work, you should be under the direct care of a qualified herbalist.

KIDNEY CLEANSE TEA

The following ingredients, combined in tea form according to the weights specified below, usually yield excellent results:

2 parts bearberry leaves (*Uva ursi*)

2 parts marshmallow root (*Althaea officinalis*)

2 parts cornsilk (*Zea mays*)

1 part dandelion leaf (*Taraxacum officinalis*)

1 part juniper berries (*Juniperus communis*)

Uva ursi is an excellent antiseptic for the whole urinary tract.

Marshmallow is soothing to the whole urinary system.

Cornsilk is also antiseptic, diuretic and anti-inflammatory to the bladder and kidneys.

Juniper berries, although not for long-term use, can clear an infection in a matter of hours. Although tincture is best, three or four berries steeped in hot water for ten minutes before drinking can very quick-acting.

HOW DO I MAKE KIDNEY CLEANSE TEA?

To make the tea, mix the herbs according to weight and add two tablespoons of the dried herbal mixture to one litre of filtered water. Soak overnight and in the morning simmer for 15 minutes. Drink one litre a day for a period of seven days when doing the kidney cleanse.

DIURETICS

Diuretics force the kidneys to increase the output of urine. There are several types, which work in different ways. Most often they are used to decrease blood pressure, treat heart disease and reduce fluid retention. They can also be prescribed for certain types of kidney failure and liver cirrhosis.

Sometimes the heart struggles to pump blood around the body. This lack of circulatory power results in fluid building up. Diuretics are prescribed to deal with this.

Diuretics frequently involve the loss of potassium, which is why the two are often prescribed together. Many herbs that have a diuretic action, such as dandelion, also contain an abundance of potassium. Dandelion is certainly the safest herbal diuretic; however, it is also important to drink plenty of water (also a diuretic) as low-level dehydration is more common than many people think. Tea made from parsley water is also a gentle diuretic that won't stress the kidneys. This can be made by adding a teaspoon of chopped parsley to a mug of hot water, and leaving it to steep for five minutes before drinking.

I believe that prescribing chemical diuretics to increase water output should be a last resort as there is a risk of overstimulating an already tired organ. Even the stronger herbal diuretics can potentially weaken the kidneys. Identification of the source of the fluid retention is therefore important.

A Western diet, high in meat and salt, puts the kidneys under great pressure. I have seen many patients' kidneys improve by dramatically reducing protein and salt consumption. Many people who overdo the protein and salt have dark rings around their eyes, which can be a symptom of sluggish kidneys. Others just have mild fluid retention, all of which respond well to a more suitable diet.

NATURAL MEDICINE AND THE KIDNEYS

In Chinese medicine the kidneys' role in health is believed to be far wider than eliminating liquid waste. The Chinese discuss other aspects of the kidneys, which from a Western point of view are probably related to the adrenal glands. The adrenal glands (discussed further in Chapter 10) sit on each kidney and provide the 'flight or fight' response to dangerous situations by producing adrenalin and noradrenalin. As well as having a regulatory effect on blood pressure, the adrenal glands also help us cope with stress by producing cortisol, which, among many actions, raises blood sugar levels to deal with an emergency. High levels of cortisol over extended periods, however, can cause muscle wastage and damage the immune system and general homeostasis, or metabolic equilibrium. The adrenal glands also produce dehydroepiandrosterone (DHEA), a substance that science knows little about other than that it is related to muscles, bones and general health. Some researchers suggest that a gradual decline in DHEA levels in the body accounts for a drop in vitality and the visible effects of ageing.

Chinese medicine states that the kidneys are also the source of heat and vitality in the body and that they relate to the emotion

THE KIDNEY FLUSH

juice of 1 lemon

juice of 1 lime (if limes are not available then use a total of 2 lemons)

½–1 tsp cayenne pepper

1 tsp maple syrup

1 glass filtered water

Prepare the kidney flush drink by shaking the ingredients together in a bottle or a jar or blend them all together. Take every morning on an empty stomach for a week. On the same day, drink 1 litre of the kidney cleanse tea (see page 193) and the barley water (see page 196).

of fear. This makes sense, given the function and positioning of the adrenal glands.

Excessive fear and anxiety, which seem to be symptoms of modern life, undermine the health of the kidney and the adrenal glands. Conversely, any weakness in these organs also gives rise to anxiety and fears.

BARLEY WATER

Barley water is especially good for you when you are cleaning out the kidneys and bladder. Barley has demulcent qualities, which means that it can reduce inflammation in the mucous membranes. Barley is also cooling, and helps clear heat from the bladder as well. It is ideal for cooling the body down on a hot day.

½ cup whole barley

6 cups water

½ stick of cinnamon

a little grated ginger

1 lemon

Simmer the ingredients together for 20 minutes. After the mixture has cooled, strain and add the fresh juice of the lemon for extra flavour and drink it throughout the day. Prepare the drink fresh each day and take it with you in a flask if you're going to be away from home.

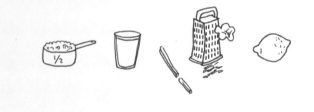

Chapter 10

LIFESTYLE

I have used the analogy of the wheel of health and the actual robustness of the wheel being related to the body type we have inherited. However, broadly speaking we are looking at the strength of the constitution. As discussed in the introduction, we all know people who live in a less than healthy way – they might smoke, drink a lot of alcohol and have taken drugs – yet live to a ripe old age. Whereas, at the other extreme, another individual might have to make a huge effort eating a good diet and looking after themselves in order to be healthy. The strength of our constitution depends on:

- our parents' health and family history

- the health and age of our parents at the time of conception

- the nutritional status and general wellbeing of our mother when we were in the womb

- whether we were breastfed

- the number of toxic factors we were exposed to in the womb and when we were growing.

Chinese medicine understands that our constitutional essence is stored in the kidneys and adrenals. This essence is difficult to define; it is, in some ways, our genetic potential.

THE ADRENAL GLANDS

The adrenal glands sit on top of the kidneys and are essential to the body's health. They excrete many important hormones and natural steroids such as adrenalin (epinephrine), DHEA, testosterone, noradrenalin and cortisol and enable the body to perform many important functions.

Adrenal exhaustion

Adrenal exhaustion is a term used in naturopathy. It is the general fatigue and lethargy experienced by people who have fought the effects of stress, usually over a long period.

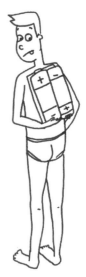

The concept of adrenal fatigue is a condition not fully recognised by Western medicine, except in the case of rare and severe adrenal disease such as with Addison's or Cushing syndrome.

Tiredness is the most common symptom among patients visiting my clinic for the first time. Now obviously, there are many causes of tiredness. Adrenal stress, however, though largely unrecognised in the orthodox medical world, is, in holistic medicine, one of the most common causes of the feeling of exhaustion. It is also the most common factor in long-term ill health.

STRESS

Have you noticed that everyone seems so much more stressed? Those working, those not working, young people, old people, parents, children, even pets. According to some recent research it seems that we are all more stressed than we used to be – the average level of stress has doubled in the last four years (AXA PPP Healthcare 2010).

We now know that stress is a big cause of disease (or 'dis-ease') – the problem is that it can creep up on us and before we know it we can have all kinds of physical, mental and emotional symptoms.

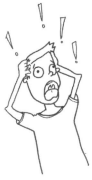

What is stress?

A dictionary definition of stress might be, 'a state of mental or emotional strain or tension resulting from adverse or very demanding circumstances'. On a day-to-day level I would define stress as 'the tension between what we want to happen and what is actually happening'.

Stress is not just an isolated mental thought process – stress is chemical. When we feel under pressure, our body produces hormones which are so powerful that they can change the way we function day-to-day. The stress hormones are produced by the adrenal glands. They produce the hormones adrenalin, noradrenalin and cortisol, which are released into the bloodstream to help us deal with an emergency. They are part of the flight or fight response. These chemical responses are only designed to be called upon infrequently, as the body has to work hard to process them and burn them up. This is usually done by literally running away. However, the kind of stress that most of us experience can be every day. We don't have the opportunity to use up the hormones, and as a result they end up accumulating in our body. We now know that the effects can be wide-reaching, from heart disease to weight gain. Mental and physical symptoms are listed below:

Mental:

- anger
- anxiety
- changes in behaviour
- depression
- difficulty concentrating
- difficulty sleeping
- feeling tired
- food cravings
- frequent crying
- lack of appetite.

Physical:

- biting your nails
- breathlessness
- chest pains
- constipation
- cramps or muscle spasms
- diarrhoea
- difficulty sleeping
- dizziness
- fainting spells, where you temporarily lose consciousness

- feeling restless

- muscular aches

- nervous twitches

- pins and needles

- sexual difficulties, such as erectile dysfunction or a loss of sexual desire

- sweating more.

The adrenals excrete hormones that help us deal with physical, emotional and biological stress. When we experience chronic stress, the constant output of hormones such as cortisol will, over time, deplete the adrenals' capacity to summon the flight or fight response. This is because, by producing cortisol over an extended period of time, they cannot create the counterbalance hormone, DHEA, in sufficient quantity.

Symptoms of adrenal fatigue are:

- underlying fatigue and exhaustion

- tiredness upon waking, even with sufficient sleep

- feeling most awake late in the evening

- poor digestion with a tendency to irritable bowel syndrome (IBS)

- a craving for stimulants and sugary foods

- poor recovery from exercise or illness

- being easily overwhelmed and/or feeling on the edge (wired)

- fluctuations in blood sugar levels

- signs of premature ageing

- illness as soon as you have a holiday or a few days off

- erratic fluctuation of blood pressure

- sudden feelings of anxiety or palpitations when attempting to relax

- vomiting when stressed.

How the body responds to stress

1. Hormones such as adrenalin are excreted into the bloodstream as part of the fight or flight response.

2. Breathing and heart rate quicken to supply more oxygen as the body prepares for action.

3. Blood vessels constrict and blood is redirected from the extremities to the brain, heart and lungs.

4. Some organ processes such as the digestive system slow down.

5. Blood becomes thicker so that any wounds will heal more quickly.

The body is designed to deal with short bursts of stress. However, over longer periods, high quantities of stress hormones begin to circulate, which can be difficult to deal with. Fatigue, heart disease, unstable blood pressure, weight gain, immune depletion, digestive disorders, cancer and osteoporosis are just a few of the conditions that this can cause.

Eventually the mechanism the body uses to regulate and produce cortisol wears out. It is then that people fail to produce *enough* cortisol. At this stage people report feeling not just wired and stressed, but completely fatigued – completely burnt out. They are often in the chronic fatigue spectrum and often have some kind of chronic condition as a result of the body being unable to control the background inflammatory factors. People then need stimulants such as caffeine and nicotine just to function.

When there is a stress factor, the body responds by releasing stress hormones which help us deal with the stressor and what it perceives as a life-threatening situation. It then attempts to return the blood chemistry back to a normal level, as the body understands that these stress hormones are toxic if they circulate for too long. If this keeps happening persistently, and if someone doesn't have the opportunity to recover sufficiently, then eventually the body gives up and no longer produces enough cortisol. Of course, depending on their genetics/constitution, nutrition and frame of mind, some people are able to cope with stress better than others.

When the adrenals get tired from being overstimulated, we tend to resort to stimulants such as caffeine to function normally. In Chinese medicine, the function of the adrenal glands is called the kidney's qi. It has been recognised from ancient times that the strength of this energy is the foundation of all health and that the most common causes of its depletion are fear, overexertion… and stress.

Sources of stress

'Pressure' on the body can be physical, mental, emotional and even spiritual. When the demands placed on the individual are greater than the internal resources available, pressure becomes 'stress'. Stress, howsoever caused, can lead to disease, and adrenal exhaustion can be at the root of most diseases.

In the twenty-first century our bodies have much to deal with: toxicity from the environment such as chemical pollution, electromagnetic radiation, poisoning from mercury fillings, root canal fillings, vaccinations – the list goes on. And, living in this world of information overload, we have developed an addiction to constant stimulation.

Our brain doesn't distinguish between emotional and physiological stress; the biochemical reactions are the same – and equally detrimental.

Mental patterns that contribute to internal stress include:

• being a perfectionist

- procrastination

- over-concern about other people's opinions

- not being able to embrace uncertainty.

When we have had traumatic events happen to us, we might develop the habit of responding to potential stress negatively. We begin anticipating danger in an inappropriately fearful way.

We all have different stress thresholds. The journey to optimum health involves knowing your limits. Watch out for feelings of being overwhelmed and make sure you get the support you need in your life. An optimistic outlook will help to combat stress; however, pretending that problems don't exist and projecting a veneer of apparent positivity is not helpful.

Dealing with stress

You can reduce stress by tackling its causes, especially those concerning relationships and finances, head on. Take action – procrastination can lead to frustration and low self-esteem.

Other action you can take to reduce stress includes:

- *Cut out caffeine, sugars, refined carbohydrates, processed foods and stimulants.* These force the adrenals into action.

- *Take vitamins and fats.* B12 is especially important for restoring the function of adrenals and is frequently deficient. Vitamin C is also important for the adrenals and can be found in vegetable juices, wheatgrass juice, rose hips, parsley, kiwi fruits, lycii berries and amla fruit (*Phyllanthus emblica*). Fats are used by the body to produce adrenal hormones. Good sources are flaxseeds, hemp seeds, avocado, coconut oil and butter.

- *Work with the natural rhythms in the body and eat at the same time each day.* There is a lot of focus on what we eat, but not enough on how and when we eat. Eating at erratic times of the day disturbs digestion, disrupts blood sugar levels and plays havoc with the adrenals.

- *Reduce the time you spend on the computer and watching TV, particularly at night.* These are stimulating activities and can affect the quality of your sleep.

- *Learn to meditate.* Methods which invoke deep relaxation will help to rest your adrenal glands. Some people are more suited to activities such as yoga and tai chi.

- If you are a perfectionist...stop it!

- *Be spontaneous.* New activities can help establish a new you. Consider taking up acting, singing, group therapy or 5-Rhythms dance.

- *Sleep it off.* Studies have shown that people who sleep less are more likely to suffer from diabetes, obesity and other chronic disorders. Most people need eight hours' sleep to be at their best, though many can only achieve six. Make sure you get the hours that you, as an individual, need. Establish a routine by going to bed and getting up at the same time each day. (Eastern medicine states that waking up before sunrise is best.) Make sure you sleep in a darkened room, which helps your brain produce the hormone 'melatonin'. Use black out blinds if necessary. This supports deep regenerative sleep, and the maintenance of a healthy weight and immune system.

> The secret of health preservation is first of all sleep. It can regenerate the essence, improve health, invigorate the spleen and stomach and strengthen the bones and muscles. (Li Yu, Qing dynasty)

- *Working with a therapist or a therapeutic group* can help identify unhealthy beliefs and provide an opportunity to release blocked emotions.

Treating stress

Acupuncture and cranial osteopathy can work directly on the nervous system and the adrenal glands. Anything relaxing will help; try deep massage and body work.

Tonic herbs (scientific name adaptogen) are very powerful herbal medicines that maintain and help restore the adrenal glands, thus helping you adapt to stress. Try:

- ashwagandha
- astragalas
- fresh oat seed
- gotu kola
- liquorice
- panax ginseng
- reishi
- rhodiola
- schisandra berry
- siberian ginseng.

More and more research is being published about the effects of adaptogens and we are starting to understand the positive impact they have on the immune, hormonal and cognitive functions.

Mineral-based medicines, such as Shilajeet from the Himalayas, are called rasayanas in Ayurveda (literally translated as the elixir of youth). They 'tonify' the body. However, they need to be made correctly and by hand. Many of these types of tonics take several months to prepare properly. At my clinic we make tonics based on ancient prescriptions originating from Indian, Chinese and Arabic medical traditions. Good quality tonic herbs, prepared correctly, can bring about a remarkable improvement in health. However, like people, herbs have different personalities, so they need to be taken according to body type.

OUR CONSTITUTION

Constitution is something that needs consideration when treating patients. Many people refer to someone as having a weak or strong constitution. So what does this mean?

In some traditions, constitution is defined as essence; something that you inherit from your parents and that to some extent defines your level of health reserve. The Chinese have the concept of jing, a substance inherent within us from birth. Reserves of jing are finite: once used up, our life force is spent and it is time to 'leave this mortal coil'. Much holistic medicine is based on the effort to preserve this essence. In traditional Greek medicine it is called original moisture and original heat. An analogy of this is Aladdin's lamp. As children, we have an abundance of original moisture and heat and the lamp burns brightly. Over time the oil begins to run out and the lamp begins to burn less brightly. Certain activities serve to deplete the reserve of oil or essence quicker than others. These are most typically:

- childbirth and raising too many children for women

- drugs (especially cocaine, ecstasy and steroids)

- excess sex and ejaculation for men

- inappropriate exercise

- insufficient rest and sleep

- overwork.

Certain factors can indicate the strength of a person's constitution. A late closing of the fontanel (soft spot on the baby's skull), weak teeth and slower development would all indicate a low jing level. The size of patients' ear lobes and the strength of their jaws are also indicators of jing reserves.

Constitutional strength is an important consideration and physicians should aim to help patients preserve their original essence. In Chinese medicine there are the qi, shen and jing.

These are our energy and life force (qi), our spirit (shen) and our constitution (jing).

The type, as well as the strength, of someone's constitution also needs to be considered. There are several ways to do this. In Ayurveda there are the three doshas: vata, pitta and kapha. Chinese medicine has five elements: water, wood, fire, earth and metal. In the traditional European medical systems there are the four temperaments – sanguine, choleric, melancholic and phlegmatic – which were widely used in Elizabethan times. Understanding your constitution makes it possible to determine the dietary, exercise and even sexual regimes that best support your physical, mental and emotional health.

Many of William Shakespeare's characters are based on the four temperaments, which have also been likened to the four suits – Hearts, Diamonds, Spades and Clubs – in playing cards. People of sanguine temperament may need different lifestyles and advice from those of melancholic temperament to achieve balance and optimum health. Clearly, the study of constitutional types is enormous and, as such, beyond the scope of this book.

No one diet will suit all people at all times. While most us know this instinctively, we can sometimes lose touch with our inner-tuition, or intuition.

> In caring for life, the wise must adapt themselves to the fluctuations of cold and heat in the four seasons, live peacefully and practice temperance in joy and anger, balance between yin and yang, strength and gentleness. Hence no outward evil can impair their health and they will enjoy long lives. (*The Yellow Emperor's Inner Classic*, 150 BCE)

As I write this I have just completed a three-day juice fast. During the process I was aware of how much our sense of wellbeing is related to not just what we eat but when we eat it, who we're with at the time and what is going on around us. All these factors have an immeasurable impact on how our diet affects our physical, mental and emotional wellbeing.

To detox is to let go. Throughout life we accumulate not only physical toxins but attitudes, perspectives and beliefs too, and begin to view the world through the filter of these ideas. Sometimes we have to let some of these ideas go. I believe we all carry long-term burdens such as feelings of anger, resentment and guilt. To let go of something is a conscious decision. And to let it go we sometimes have to experience it consciously.

Case history: Letting go of resentment

A patient of mine, while undergoing the liver flush, became aware of an immense resentment that would surface repeatedly during the process. The resentment was targeted at feelings that he had never voiced and included negative feelings towards his wife and his job. Only now was his body processing emotions that he had until now suppressed. During the cleanse these feelings became overwhelming, so I asked him to draw a picture of them. He produced a drawing of a dark and gloomy landscape with a small figure of a man, representing himself. Throughout the flush, these feelings of resentment and gloominess would come and go. The patient noticed, however, that by confronting the frustration and sadness, he would feel more energetic and better connected with the people around him. By letting go of the resentment he created room for connection and joy again.

If we can't get angry, we can't get enthusiastic and passionate. If we can't be sad, we cannot feel happiness. Watch children; see how they express a whole array of emotions – sadness, despair, frustration, anger, joy and excitement – often seamlessly and within a matter of minutes. This is how to be connected with life.

When we say things like, 'I shouldn't be feeling this,' or, 'I must be a bad person because I feel anger,' we suppress the feeling and prevent ourselves from expressing anger and moving on. In Chinese medicine energy, or qi, is healthy so long as it is flowing. Problems, such as sickness and depression, arise once energy becomes stagnant. Or, as someone once said to me, 'Depression is anger without enthusiasm.'

The idea that the mind and body are separate is barely a hundred years old. Ancient wisdom tells us that every organ in the body is connected with certain emotions. People would describe themselves as liverish if they felt sluggish and depressed, or would 'vent their spleen' when angry.

Sometimes, getting better presents new challenges. I remember someone speaking of the terror he felt because he was recovering from an illness he had had all his life. Now he was creating a new life, complete with new relationships, work and other activities previously unavailable to him. Sometimes when we find wellness we also have to find aspects of ourselves that have lain dormant.

Chapter 11

ACTIVATION

EXERCISE AND PHYSICAL ACTIVITY

> Nurturing life requires that one keep oneself as fluid as possible. One should not stay still for too long, nor should one exhaust oneself by trying to perform impossible tasks. One should learn how to exercise from nature, by observing the fact that flowing water never stagnates and a busy door with active hinges never rusts or rots. Why? Because they exercise themselves perpetually and are almost always moving. (Sun Simiao, seventh century AD)

Activation is an exceedingly important aspect to being truly well. Although I only briefly touch on it in this book, it is essential to value the importance of movement in keeping healthy and becoming healthy.

Most of us in the Western world do not move enough. Exercise has become synonymous merely with weight loss and, while it is important to maintain a healthy weight, it is only one of its many benefits. Exercise benefits us physically, mentally, emotionally and spiritually.

What is exercise?

The World Health Organization (WHO 2011) says, 'Physical activity is defined as any bodily movement produced by skeletal muscles that requires energy expenditure.'

What does exercise do?

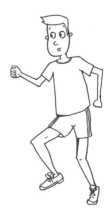

- *Improves the immune system.* Regular exercise makes us less likely to suffer from colds and flu as well as degenerative disorders such as cancer.

- *Lowers cholesterol.* More important than just reducing the overall cholesterol level, exercise improves the ratio of good to bad fats.

- *Improves existing conditions* such as arthritis, cancer, osteoporosis and many others.

- *Helps prevent disease* such as diabetes, depression and Alzheimer's. Seven hours of brisk walking every week has been shown to lower the rates of colon-rectal cancer rates by 40 per cent (Halle and Schoenberg 2009). Up to a third of breast cancer cases could be avoided if women from developing countries took more exercise (La Vecchia 2010).

- *Improves your mood.* Because of the effect it has on your endorphins, exercise can help your mood and combat depression and anxiety.

- *Prevents strokes.* Research has shown that exercise reduces the risk of suffering and dying from a stroke by 27 per cent and cuts the risk of a cerebral haemorrhage in men by 40 per cent (Reimers, Knapp and Reimers 2009).

- *Releases frustration, tension and anger.*

IF YOU REST, YOU RUST!

The vast majority of us do not move or exercise enough. The WHO recommends that adults undertake at least 30 minutes of moderate physical activity at least five times a week. This is considered the minimum for basic health. Children are advised to partake in 60 minutes of moderate to vigorous activity every day. Unfortunately, it seems that as countries develop and become more affluent, their populations take less exercise and die of more chronic diseases arising from sedentary and stagnant lifestyles. It is estimated that 1.9 million deaths around the world every year are attributed to lack of physical activity (WHO 2011).

In cultures such as the Maasai of Kenya, where there is very little chronic disease, there are no gyms or structured exercise regimes. Instead, people keep active in their day-to-day lives by collecting water, preparing meals, herding cows, and so on.

In embracing modern conveniences we have become inactive. Now, I'm not saying we should throw away our washing machines and only collect well water in order to be healthy, but we do need to be active every day. Movement and activity need to be part of our day, whether we are working or not.

Good ways to stay active in the modern world are walking to work – or parking further away if you have to drive – and using stairs instead of lifts and escalators and taking a walk after lunch. Growing vegetables and other forms of gardening are also great exercise.

I remember talking to an owner of a gym who said his profits came from people who took up membership, but hardly attended. The majority of his membership fell into this category – including me. If you decide to join a gym, a personal trainer could also help you maintain your motivation and get your money's worth. Alternatively, organised classes such as spinning or aerobics provide excellent cardiovascular exercise for people with busy lifestyles. Other forms of exercise worth considering are:

- *Swimming.* A great way to build stamina and move the body without putting strain on the joints. Be sure to wash the chlorine off your body afterwards.

- *Cycling.* Also great for building stamina and moving the body. The circular movement is conducive to energy flow without it jarring the body.

- *Yoga.* A fantastic way to build health. The stretching will increase the flow of qi and strengthen your inner core.

- *Dancing.* Whatever style you choose, dancing is excellent exercise. I like five-rhythms which unblocks stagnant qi. Also, you don't need to 'look good' – or be able to dance!

- *Tai chi and qi gong.* These build inner resources and train the mind.

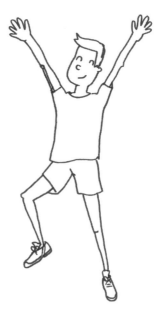

Exercise from the Eastern traditions are based on developing your inner qi and energy, thus building your inner reserves. I have seen patients who have developed their muscles but failed to build inner strength – they look good but lack the protective health benefits provided by internal exercises such as yoga, tai chi and qi gong.

TOO MUCH…OR TOO LITTLE?

Although rare, it is possible to over-exercise. You can see evidence of this in some athletes who train excessively when younger, then reach their thirties feeling exhausted. Sadly, many of these people also die young. I often see this in cases of gymnasts who, having trained rigorously while going through puberty, have gone on to have difficulties with menstruation, fertility and vitality.

People who over-train tend to get frequent injuries or develop chronic problems which do not heal. They can also become more susceptible to illness and infection as their inner reserves get used up.

Chapter 12

MIND, EMOTIONS AND SPIRIT

EMOTIONS AND HOW THEY CAN CREATE DISEASE

Holistic medicine places great emphasis on emotions and their effect on health and disease; it recognises the strong connection between the emotional, mental and physical aspects of the self. If there is disharmony on the emotional and mental level, it will undoubtedly manifest on the physical, and vice versa. For example, with excessive alcohol intake and damage to the liver, a person may be prone to anger and irritation. Similarly, long-term irritation also affects the flow of qi through the liver and, ultimately, its physical function.

Difficult events in life can give rise to illness. The Life Stress Inventory, created in 1967 by two psychiatrists, Holmes and Rahe, examined 5000 medical records to determine whether stressful life events and subsequent illnesses were linked. They created a scoring system, allocating points to each stressful event. Points were allocated according to how stressful an event was considered. Holmes and Rahe found that that there was indeed a correlation between the experiencing of stressful events and the occurrence of illness within 12 months.

Furthermore, when Holmes and Rahe conducted cross-cultural studies, the results were the same, suggesting that the link between stressful events and physical health is universal.

Their top ten stressful life events are:

1. Spouse's death.

2. Divorce.

3. Marriage separation.

4. Jail term.

5. Death of a close relative.

6. Injury or illness.

7. Marriage.

8. Losing one's job.

9. Marriage reconciliation.

10. Retirement.

Stress is a word that many of us use to describe uncomfortable feelings. It has become a recent trend in medicine to classify any emotional or mental strain as stress. Accordingly, many current medical studies have attributed a multitude of symptoms to stress. Although these symptoms can be attributed to other problems too, an increasing number of studies are confirming the link between our mental and emotional state and our physical wellbeing. (See also the section on stress on page 198.)

Ancient physicians, over years of observation, have noticed how certain emotions and thoughts have created disharmony in certain organs. Similarly a disharmony in an organ can also give rise to certain mental or emotional states.

This concept of emotion/disease connection goes beyond stress but makes the connection between, say, fear and its effects on the kidney and adrenal glands.

The Life Stress Inventory demonstrates that certain events have an impact on wellbeing. However, I don't believe we can define our mental and emotional health so simply. Stress can describe many feelings – irritation, frustration, negativity, depression, grief, betrayal and fear, to name just a few. We need a language that can describe how we feel because, often, simply being able to identify an uncomfortable feeling is enough for its impact to subside and be released.

HOW DO EMOTIONS CAUSE DISEASE?

Events in our lives are not, of themselves, the cause of disease; our emotional responses and how we, as individuals, view those events provide the link between an occurrence and an illness. One person may feel sadness and grief about bereavement; another may feel relief or even anger. Each can trigger differing physical reactions.

Our minds and bodies are in constant communication. When we have any emotional and mental activity our brain produces neuropeptides, which means our cells are always aware of how we are thinking and feeling. Recurring feelings and thoughts, then, will surely create an energetic imprint in our bodies. So what will be the physical impact of frequent bouts of anxiety, irritation or sadness?

The Chinese see a correlation between emotions and areas of the body. They use an analogy of qi, or vital force, as a living substance that connects and flows through our body, mind and psyche. It's like water; as long as it flows unhindered it will remain clean and healthy. However, if the water is interrupted on its course it will become stagnant. In the same way an emotional pattern of anger will create an imbalance, resulting in a physical disease.

Emotions in themselves are neither good nor bad. They are all necessary parts of our human experience. When emotions flow easily and appropriately it gives rise to better physical harmony.

In Chinese medicine, emotional causes of disease are referred to as 'internal causes of disease', with each major emotion linked to organs in the body. They are:

- anger and frustration – liver

- anxiety and fear – kidneys and adrenals

- sadness and grief – lungs

- joy or lack of joy – heart

- over-thinking and worry – stomach and the digestive system.

Fear

Anxiety and fear, over a period of time, as mentioned, will wear out our adrenal glands. In turn, when the adrenals are on a high state of alert, we experience further feelings of anxiety, meaning that we interpret our life experiences in a more fearful way.

Fear is the emotion we experience when we think something bad is going to happen. It arises when we anticipate impending danger or a negative experience such as pain.

Like any emotion, fear can be excessive or insufficient. When a person is out of balance they can either take lots of risks and feel no fear at all, or become consumed by fear and rendered unable to do anything.

Some people may experience fear when there is no obvious threat. This can happen if the person has had an experience, such as a road accident, that evoked strong feelings. It may be classed as post-traumatic stress syndrome: the threat may have passed but the feelings of fear are still present.

Balanced correctly, however, fear is an extremely important emotion. Anyone who has walked with young children who have suddenly run towards a busy road will know that feeling of panic and horror – and the surge of adrenalin – all too well. This flight and fight response enables us to act quickly and instinctively to prevent the child from being in danger. Such balanced fear is appropriate and acts as a vital tool for our protection and that of others.

Fear usually compels us to take action. It is future orientated and once the situation has passed the feeling of fear and anxiety usually goes.

Shock

A shock is a sudden unexpected, upsetting experience. Most of us have experienced shock at some point. Shock can be felt indirectly, such as learning of a death or a disaster, or directly, such as being attacked. Shock is also subjective: learning of a pregnancy could be a wonderful event for one person – a shock to another.

Unlike fear, shock blocks and freezes the flow of qi and energy. Trauma can get stuck in the body, a symptom I often see with patients who experienced birth trauma. While they cannot remember the birth itself, the trauma has left physical, mental and emotional effects. Once this trapped energy is released, qi floods the body and psyche.

Good ways to release trapped trauma in the body are:

- massage

- EMDR (Eye Movement Desensitisation and Re-processing), a form of psychotherapy that helps to resolve the effects of traumatic experiences. The process, which usually involves the eye and movements, helps to release distress that has been stored in the body and nervous system

- EFT (Emotional Freedom Technique), a technique of stimulating acupuncture points, which can help to release blocked emotions trapped in the energy system of the body

- dancing.

Anger

> Anger: a strong feeling of annoyance, displeasure, or hostility. (New Oxford Dictionary of English)

Feelings of anger can encompass a whole spectrum of sensations and are often regarded as destructive and negative. When you think of anger you may imagine acts of violence, shouting, even rape and murder. Anger can be intense and highly destructive.

However, healthy and appropriate expression of anger can also be a vital part of our wellbeing and, I believe, physical health. Anger arises when our boundaries are transgressed. So, if we feel under attack, anger will help us to protect ourselves.

To be human is to feel all emotions. Some are more uncomfortable than others, but none are inherently good or bad. We restrict, suppress and repress our feelings, usually by judging them. Anger allows for growth, change and challenge.

CHANNELLING ANGER

> Anyone can become angry – that is easy. But to be angry with the right person, to the right degree, at the right time, for the right purpose, and in the right way; this is not easy. (Aristotle, quoted in Goleman 2006)

If we don't feel anger and express it healthily, then it can easily turn into frustration, inertia and even depression.

When I was writing this chapter, I came across a workshop called 'How to control your anger'. I think it should be 'How to channel your anger'. Physical exercise is probably one of the most effective ways to transform and release tension, frustration and anger.

Joy

Our natural state is to be joyful. In Vedic Indian philosophy, it is said that our soul is naturally in a state of Sat (truth), Cit (consciousness) and Ananda (bliss). This means that our natural state is that we are situated in bliss and knowledge. However, for most of us, joy is related to experience.

I think there is an obsession in the West with being happy. Surely to be human is to feel sadness, anger, fear and joy, appropriately?

The Chinese believe excessive joy is a cause of disease. I personally don't come across a lot of people who are ill from experiencing too much joy. Another interpretation could be over-stimulation, of which we have a huge amount of input from our environment. Overstimulation can burn up our qi and deplete our essence.

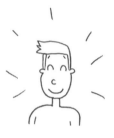

Sadness and grief

Grief is caused by the loss of something – or someone – cherished. It is probably the most difficult of all emotions to process. We can feel grief for anything we once were connected to such as:

- a loved one

- a pet

- dreams and aspirations

- possessions, such as our home

- a child who leaves home (empty nest syndrome)

- a relationship.

The psychotherapist Dr Elisabeth Kübler-Ross has written extensively about the process of grieving. She refers to the grief cycle, which encompasses commonly felt emotions such as denial, anger, bargaining, depression and acceptance. Grief is individual – how we deal with it is personal to us – though it does mean letting go of hopes and dreams.

> Give sorrow words; the grief that does not speak whispers the o'er-fraught heart and bids it break. (William Shakespeare, *Macbeth*, Act IV, scene III)

In Chinese medicine, it is said that grief is connected with the lungs and our immune system.

RITUAL

All cultures deal with loss and grief in different ways; however, ritual is frequently part of the process. If you feel that you are still holding onto grief, find a ritual that will help you to let it go. One example might be to write a letter to a person that you've lost, take it to a local river and let it go. Another idea is to create a list of your sources of grief, then ceremoniously burn it.

Case history: Grief

'After my dad died I noticed that I had a cough. It lasted for months and months, and although I had medical check-ups, they could find nothing. It was then that I looked into what else it could be. I went to an acupuncturist who detected a disharmony on my pulses which, they said, can reflect stuck grief that was impacting on my lungs. I had an acupuncture treatment to strengthen my lungs and help me to let go. The effects hit me the next day. All I could do was cry for a day or two. I was shocked by the amount of sadness within me, and realised that I hadn't taken enough time to really let go of my dad. Although I still get episodes of feeling sad, I feel that it is no longer stuck within me and creating physical problems. The cough also cleared up in a week or two.'

Accepting that we need help is a big step forward in dealing with grief.

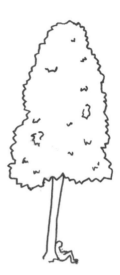

THE WHEEL TURNS

To be healthy we need to flow in rhythm with our natural cycle. If we are in tune with our own wheel of health, we can encounter harsh terrain – the unforeseen bumps and dips in the road – and still remain balanced. As long as we steadily encourage our body's natural equilibrium through how we live, what we eat, how we move and think, we will maintain a good level of health with very little conscious effort.

I feel that modern medicine can take us on a detour which is based on dealing with symptoms. In many ways it seems to have bypassed the most important factor in regaining true health… the cause.

Ancient medicine is based around the two things I feel are the most important when dealing with improving health as well as illness and dis-ease. That is the individual, and the cause of their illness. No two people are alike. No single diet will be good for everyone. We have to consider why we have become ill, not just treat the symptom.

Which takes us back to the wheel of health:

- *Genetics.* Understanding what our constitution is and how we can work with it.

- *Environment.* What are we exposing ourselves to and how to make the best of it.

- *Nourishment.* How we can support our body by consciously choosing what's best to put in it.

- *Detoxification.* Encouraging the body to eliminate unwanted toxins.

- *Lifestyle.* Choosing a way of life tailored to our body's needs.

- *Activation.* Moving our body in the way it needs to prevent stagnation.

- *Mind, emotions and spirit.* Supporting our non-physical parts.

- *The centre of the wheel.* A place of balance and equilibrium.

Our individuality makes us who we are, and so illness will express itself in a different way from person to person. Each of us needs to be treated in a slightly different way, because the disharmony often stems from a different cause.

And so, to move toward heath you must know yourself, you must know your nature. Because it's that nature which keeps the wheel turning, in a moment by moment striving to…make yourself better…

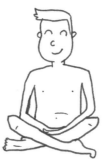

REFERENCES

Allen, F. (1915) 'Prolonged fasting in diabetes.' *American Journal of the Medical Sciences 150*, 480–485.

American Academy of Periodontology (2011) 'Gum Disease Links to Heart Disease and Strokes.' Available at www.perio.org/consumer/mbc.heart.htm, accessed on 18 October 2011.

Arrieta, M.C., Bistritz, L. and Meddings, J.B. (2006) 'Alterations in intestinal permeability.' *Gut 55*, 1512–1520.

Ascherio, A., Katan, M.B., Zock, P.L., Stampfer, M.J. and Willett, W.C. (1999) 'Trans fatty acids and coronary heart disease.' *New England Journal of Medicine 340*, 25, 1994–1998.

AXA PPP Healthcare (2010) 'Stress Management.' Available at www.axappphealthcare.co.uk/uk-business/business-resource-centre/features/stress-management, accessed on 29 October 2011.

Baker, B.P., Benbrook, C.M., Groth III, E. and Lutz Benbrook, K. (2002) 'Pesticide residues in conventional, IPM-grown and organic foods: Insights from three U.S. data sets.' *Food Additives and Contaminants 19*, 5, 427–446.

BBC (2010) 'Obese children show signs of heart disease.' Available at news.bbc.co.uk/1/hi/health/8538426.stm, accessed on 11 August 2011.

Benbrook, C., Zhao, X., Yanez, J., Davies, N. and Andrews, P. (2008) *New Evidence Confirms the Nutritional Superiority of Plant-Based Organic Foods.* State of Science Review, March. Boulder, CO: The Organic Center.

Benke, G., Abramson, M., Raven, J., Thien, F.C.K. and Walters, E.H. (2004) 'Asthma and vaccination history in a young adult cohort.' *Australian and New Zealand Journal of Public Health 28*, 336–338.

Black, C.D., Herring, M.P., Hurley, D.J. and O'Connor, P.J. (2010) 'Ginger (Zingiber officinale) reduces muscle pain caused by eccentric exercise.' *The Journal of Pain 11*, 9, 894–903.

Blaylock, R.L. (1994) *Excitotoxins: The Taste That Kills.* Santa Fe, NM: Health Press.

Bolland, M.J., Grey, A., Avenall, A., Gamble, G.D. and Reid, I.R.(2011) 'Calcium supplements with or without vitamin D and risk of cardiovascular events: reanalysis of the Women's Health Initiative limited access dataset and meta-analysis.' *British Journal of Medicine 342*: d2040.

Bragg, P. (2004) *The Miracle of Fasting*, 5th edition. Santa Barbara, CA: Health Science and Live Products.

Brown, S.E. (2000) *Better Bones, Better Body.* Columbus, OH: McGraw-Hill Contemporary.

Butler, G., Nielsen, J H., Slots, T., Seal, C., Eyre, M. D., Sanderson, R. and Leifert, C. (2008) 'Fatty acid and fat-soluble antioxidant concentrations in milk from high- and low-input conventional and organic systems: seasonal variation.' *Journal of the Science of Food and Agriculture 88*, 1431–1441.

Buttram, H.E. (2000) 'Vaccine Scene 2000 – Review and Update.' *Medical Sentinel* March/ April. Association of American Physicians and Surgeons.

Carlo, G. and Schram, M. (2001) *Cell Phones: Invisible Hazards in the Wireless Age: An Insider's Alarming Discoveries About Cancer and Genetic Damage.* New York: Carroll & Graf Publishers.

Centre for Disease Control and Prevention (2010) 'Vaccine Excipient and Media Summary, Part 2.' Available at www.cdc.gov/vaccines/vac-gen/additives.htm, accessed on 29 November 2011.

Christopher, J.R. (1976) *School of Natural Healing.* Springville, UT: Christopher Publications.

Clark, T. J. (2007) 'Soil Mineral Depletion.' Available at www.tjclark.co.nz/jurassic_soil.htm, accessed on 29 November 2011.

Cousins, B. (2000a) *Cooking Without.* London: Thorsons.

Cousins, B. (2000b) *Vegetarian Cooking Without.* London: Thorsons.

Cox, I.M., Campbell, M.J. and Dowson, D. (1991) 'Red blood cell magnesium and chronic fatigue syndrome.' *Lancet 337*, 8744, 757–760.

Drasch, G., Schupp, I., Höfl, H., Reinke, R. and Roider, G. (1994) 'Mercury burden of human fetal and infant tissues.' *European Journal of Pediatrics 153*, 8, 607–610. Available at dx.doi.org/10.1007/BF02190671, accessed on 18 October 2011.

EJF (2007) *The Deadly Chemicals in Cotton.* London: Environmental Justice Foundation in collaboration with Pesticide Action Network UK.

Ellis, K., Innocent, G., Grover-White, D., Cripps, P., McLean, W.G., Howard, C.V. and Mihm, M. (2006) 'Comparing the fatty acid composition of organic and conventional milk.' *Journal of Dairy Science 89*, 1938–1950.

European Trade Union Institute (2009) 'Cancer risks: environment a "huge" factor.' Available at http://hesa.etui-rehs.org/uk/newsevents/newsfiche.asp?pk=1265, accessed on 11 August 2011.

Foodconsumer (2010) 'Studies explain why girls enter puberty as young as age 7.' Available at www.foodconsumer.org/newsite/Nutrition/Food/girls_puberty_1008100921.html, accessed on 11 August 2011.

Freni, S.C. (1994) 'Exposure to high fluoride concentrations in drinking water is associated with decreased birth rates.' *Journal of Toxicology and Environmental Health 42*, 1, 109–121.

Gerson, C. and Walker, M. (2001) *The Gerson Therapy.* New York: Kensington Publishing.

Gerson, M. (1990) *A Cancer Therapy: Results of Fifty Cases.* San Diego, CA: The Gerson Institute.

Goleman, D. (2006) *Emotional Intelligence.* New York: Bantam Books.

Guelpa, G. (1910) 'Starvation and purgation in the relief of diabetes.' *BMJ 24*, ii, 1050–1051.

Halle, M. and Schoenberg, M.H. (2009) 'Physical activity in the prevention and treatment of colorectal carcinoma.' *Deutsches Aerzteblatt International 106*, 44, 722–726.

Hicks, A., Hicks, J. and Mole, P. (2004) *Five Element Constitutional Medicine.* London: Churchill Livingstone.

Higdon, J. (2003) 'Micronutrient Information Center: Vitamin B12.' Linus Pauling Institute at Oregon State University. Available at http://lpi.oregonstate.edu/infocenter/vitamins/vitaminB12, accessed on 6 December 2011.

Imamura, M. and Tung, T. (1984) 'A trial of fasting cure for PCB poisoned patients in Taiwan.' *American Journal of Industrial Medicine 5*, 147–153.

Jeffreys, T. (1999) *Your Health at Risk.* Hammersmith: Thorsons.

Khan, M.S. (1986) *Islamic Medicine.* London: Routledge & Kegan Paul.

Khan, A., Safdar, M., Ali Khan, M.M., Khattak, K.N. and Anderson, R.A. (2003) 'Cinnamon improves glucose and lipids of people with type 2 diabetes.' *Diabetes Care 26*, 3215–3218.

Kjeldsen-Kragh, J., Haugen, M., Borchgrevink, C.F., Laerum, E. *et al.* (1991) 'Controlled trial of fasting and one-year vegetarian diet in rheumatoid arthritis.' *Lancet*, 899–904.

Koscielny, J., Klüendorf, D., Latza, R., Schmitt, R. *et al.* (1999) 'The antiatherosclerotic effect of Allium sativum.' *Atherosclerosis 144*, 237–249.

La Vecchia, C. (2010) Figures cited from the International Agency for Research on Cancer at the European Breast Cancer Conference in Barcelona, March 2010.

Larre, C. and Rochat de la Vallee, E. (1987) (trans.) *The Yellow Emperor's Classic of Internal Medicine.* Cambridge: Monkey Press.

Lennox, W. and Cobb, S. (1928) 'Studies in Epilepsy.' *Archives of Neurology and Psychiatry 20*, 711–779.

Lu,Y., Sun, Z.R., Wu, L.N., Wang, X., Lu, W. and Liu, S.S. (2000) 'Effect of high fluoride water on intelligence in children.' *Fluoride 33*, 2, 74–78.

Mason, P. (1994) 'Calculations of American Deaths Caused by Magnesium Deficiency, as Projected from International Data.' Available at www.mgwater.com/calcs. shtml#summary, accessed on 18 October 2011.

Mendelsohn, R.S. (1993) *How to Raise a Healthy Child.* New York: Ballantine Books Inc.

Morris, M.C., Evans, D.A., Bienias, J.L., Tangney, C.C. *et al.* (2003) 'Dietary fats and the risk of incident Alzheimer disease.' *Archives of Neurology 60*, 2, 194–200.

Myhill, S. (2009) 'Heartburn – at last I have sussed out why this is such a common problem!' Available at www.drmyhill.co.uk/wiki/Heartburn_-_at_last_I_have_sussed_out_why_ this_is_such_a_common_problem!, accessed on 12 August 2011.

National Health Service (2010) 'Symptoms of stress.' Available at www.nhs.uk/Conditions/ Stress/Pages/Symptoms.aspx, accessed on 15 August 2011.

National Research Council (2006) *Fluoride in Drinking Water: A Scientific Review of EPA's Standards.* Washington, DC: National Academies Press.

Office of Pesticide Programs (2007) *Pesticides: Topical & Chemical Fact Sheets.* Washington, DC: US EPA.

Olney, J.W., Farber, N.B., Spitznagel, E. and Robins, L.N. (1986) 'Increasing brain tumor rates: is there a link to aspartame?' *Journal of Neuropathology and Experimental Neurology 55*, 11, 1115–1123.

Ortiz-Pérez, D., Rodríguez-Martínez, M., Martínez, F., Borja-Aburto, V.H., Castelo, J., Grimaldo, J.I., de la Cruz, E., Carrizales, L., Díaz-Barriga, F. (2003) 'Fluoride-induced disruption of reproductive hormones in men.' *Environmental Research 93*, 1, 20–30.

Petersen, I. and Hayward, A.C. (2007) 'Antibacterial prescribing in primary care.' *Journal of Antimicrobial Chemotherapy 60*, suppl 1, i43–i47.

Plengvidhya, V., Breidt, F. Jr, Lu, Z. and Fleming, H.P. (2007) 'DNA fingerprinting of lactic acid bacteria in sauerkraut fermentations.' *Applied and Environmental Microbiology 73*, 23, 7697–7702.

Prüss-Üstün, A. and Corvalán, C. (2006) *Preventing Disease Through Healthy Environments: Towards an estimate of the environmental burden of disease.* Geneva: World Health Organization.

Racz, K., Feher, J., Csomos, G., Varga, I., Kiss, R. and Glaz, E. (1990) 'An antioxidant drug, silibinin, modulates steroid secretion in human pathological adrenocortical cells.' *Journal of Endocrinology 124*, 341–345.

Reilly, H.J. and Hagy Brod, R. (2008) *The Edgar Cayce Handbook for Health Through Drugless Therapy.* Virginia Beach, VA: ARE Press.

Reimers, C.D., Knapp, G. and Reimers, A.K. (2009) 'Exercise as stroke prophylaxis.' *Deutsches Aertzeblatt International 106*, 44, 715–721.

Rooney, P.J., Jenkins, R.T. and Buchanan, W.W. (1990) 'A short review of the relationship between intestinal permeability and inflammatory joint disease.' *Clinical and Experimental Rheumatology 8*, 1, 75–83.

Sears, C.L. (2006) 'A dynamic partnership: Celebrating our gut flora.' *Anaerobe 12*, 2, 114.

Seeger, M. (1972) 'Soviet Cure-All: Eat Nothing for 30 Days.' *Los Angeles Times*, 3 April.

Servan-Schreiber, D. (2009) *Anticancer: A New Way of Life*. New York: Viking Adult.

Slutsky, I., Abumaria, N., Wu, L.-J., Huang, C., Zhang, L., Li, B., Zhao, X., Govindarajan, A., Zhao, M.-G., Zhuo, M., Tonegawa, S. and Liu, G. (2010) 'Enhancement of Learning and Memory by Elevating Brain Magnesium.' *Neuron 65*, 2, 165–177.

Smith, J.D., Terpening, C.M., Schmidt, S.O. and Gums, J.G. (2001) 'Relief of fibromyalgia symptoms following discontinuation of dietary excitotoxins.' *Annals of Pharmacotherapy 35*, 6, 702–706.

Stahlhut, R.W., van Wijngaarden, E., Dye, T.D., Cook, S. and Swan, S.H. (2007) 'Concentrations of urinary phthalate metabolites are associated with increased waist circumference and insulin resistance in adult U.S. males.' *Environmental Health Perspectives 115*, 6, 876–882.

Stewart, W. and Fleming, L.W. (1973) 'Features of a successful therapeutic fast of 382 days duration.' *Postgraduate Medical Journal 49*, 203–209.

Stockholm Convention (2011) 'Stockholm Convention: At a Glance.' Available at http://chm.pops.int/Portals/0/download.aspx?d=UNEP-POPS-PAWA-OVERV-AtaGlance.En.pdf, accessed on 29 November 2011.

Szekely, E.B. (1981) *The Essene Gospel of Peace*. London: International Biogenic Society.

Tenpenny, S. (2008) *Saying No to Vaccines*. Cleveland, OH: Tenpenny Publishing.

Thomas, D.E. (2003) 'A study of the mineral depletion of foods available to us as a nation over the period 1940 to 1991.' *Nutrition and Health 17*, 85–115.

Tucker, K.L., Morita, K., Qiao, N., Hannan, M.T., Cupples, L.A. and Kiel, D.P. (2006) 'Colas, but not other carbonated beverages, are associated with low bone mineral density in older women: The Framingham Osteoporosis Study.' *American Journal of Clinical Nutrition 84*, 4, 936–942.

Waring, R. (2004) 'Absorption of magnesium sulphate through the skin.' School of Biosciences, University of Birmingham (republished by the Epsom Salt Council).

Waring, R.H. (n.d.) 'Sulfate and Sulfation.' Available at www.epsomsaltcouncil.org/articles/Sulfation_Benefits_072204.pdf, accessed on 14 August 2011.

Weisinger, J.R and Bellorin-Font, E. (1998) 'Magnesium and phosphorus.' *Lancet 352*, 391–396.

WHO (2011) 'Physical Activity.' Available at www.who.int/entity/dietphysicalactivity/pa/en/index.html, accessed on 15 August 2011.

Woese, K., Lange, D., Boess, C. and Bogl, K.W. (1997) 'A comparison of organically and conventionally grown foods: results of a review of the relevant literature.' *Journal of Science, Food and Agriculture 74*, 281–293.

Woodruff, T.J., Zota, A.R. and Schwartz, J.M. (2011) 'Environmental chemicals in pregnant women in the United States: NHANES 2003–2004.' *Environmental Health Perspectives 119*, 6, 878–885.

Worthington, V. (2001) 'Nutritional quality of organic versus conventional fruits, vegetables, and grains.' *Journal Of Alternative and Complementary Medicine 7*, 2, 161–173.

Wu, M., Atchley, D., Greer, L., Janssen, S., Rosenberg, D. and Sass, J. (2009) 'Dosed Without Prescription: Preventing Pharmaceutical Contamination of Our Nation's Drinking Water.' Available at http://docs.nrdc.org/health/files/hea_10012001a.pdf, accessed on 7 November 2011.

Wurtman, R. (1983) 'Neurochemical changes following high-dose aspartame with dietary carbohydrates.' *New England Journal of Medicine 309*, 7, 429–430.

Yablokov, A.V. (2009) *Chernobyl: Consequences of the catastrophe for people and the environment*. Annals of the New York Academy of Sciences, Volume 1181. New York: New York Academy of Sciences.

Zhao, F., Wang, L. and Liu, K. (2009) 'In vitro anti-inflammatory effects of arctigenin, a lignan from Arctium lappa L., through inhibition on iNOS pathway.' *Journal of Ethnopharmacology 122*, 3, 457–462.

FURTHER READING

Alexander, K. (2007) *Dietary Healing*. Belair, South Australia: Annexus Pty Ltd.

Bartram, T. (1995) *Encyclopaedia of Herbal Medicine*. Christchurch, Dorset: Grace Publishers.

Brandt, K. and Leifert, C. (2005) 'Which aspects of health are likely to be affected by our choice of food quality, such as organic food, and how can we investigate this question?' Organic Farming Conference, 'Navigating in a new era', SLU, Ultuna, Sweden, 22–23 November 2005, pp.240–243.

Bridges, L. (2003) *Face Reading in Chinese Medicine*. Philadelphia, PA: Churchill Livingstone.

Campion, K. (1995) *The Family Medical Herbal*. London: Leopard Books.

Chaitow, L. (1996) *Principles of Fasting*. London: Thorsons.

Cott, A., Agel, J. and Boe, E. (1997) *Fasting: The Ultimate Diet*. Winter Park, FL: Hastings House/Daytrips Publishers.

Hoffer, A. (1999) *Orthomolecular Treatment for Schizophrenia*. Springfield, IL: Keats.

Holford, P. (2004) *The New Optimum Nutrition Bible*. London: Piatkus.

Kastner, J. (2004) *Chinese Nutritional Therapy*. Stuttgart: Thieme.

Katz, S. (2003) *Wild Fermentation*. Vermont: Chelsea Green Publishing Co.

Kirkman, M.F. (2002) *The Digestive Contract, Intestinal Microbiology and Probiotics*. Kent: Biopathica Ltd.

Krohn, J. and Taylor, F. (2000) *Natural Detoxification*. Vancouver: Hartley & Marks.

Lipski, E. (2004) *Digestive Wellness*. New York: Mc Graw Hill.

Macallan, S. (1999) *The Mercury Papers*. Available at www.stephenmacallan.co.uk/mercury.htm, accessed on 29 November 2011.

McCance, R.A. and Widdowson, E.M. (1960) *The Chemical Composition of Foods*, 3rd Edition. Special Report Series No. 297. London: Medical Research Council.

McCance, R.A. and Widdowson (2002) *The Composition of Foods*, 6th Edition. London: Royal Society of Chemistry/Food Standards Agency.

Montignac, M. (2010) *Glycemic Index Diet*. Monaco: Alpen Editions.

Moritz, A. (2000) *The Amazing Liver Cleanse*. Vancouver: Namaste Publishing.

Pacholok, S.M. and Stuart, J.J. (2005) *Could it be B12? An Epidemic of Misdiagnoses*. Fresno, CA: Quill Driver Books.

Peck, M.S. (1978) *The Road Less Traveled: A New Psychology of Love, Traditional Values and Spiritual Growth*. New York: Simon & Schuster.

Pitchford, P. (2002) *Healing with Whole Foods: Asian Traditions and Modern Nutrition*. Berkeley, CA: North Atlantic Books.

Phillips, A. (1999) *Dispelling Vaccination Myths.* Amherst, NY: Prometheus.

Schimmel, H.W. (1997) *Functional Medicine.* Heidelberg: Haug.

Svoboda, R.E. (1988) *Prakriti: Your Ayurvedic Constitution.* Albuquerque, NM: Geocom.

Svoboda, R.E. (2004) *Ayurveda: Life, Health and Longevity.* Alberquerque, NM: The Ayurvedic Healing Press.

Tierra, M. (1988) *Planetary Herbology.* Sante Fe, NM: Lotus Press.

Turner, R. (1990) *Naturopathic Medicine.* Wellingborough: Thorsons.

Vogel, A. (1990) *The Nature Doctor.* Edinburgh: Mainstream Publishing.

Winston, D. (2007) *Adaptogens.* Rochester, Vermont: Healing Arts Press.

RESOURCES

All About Natural Medicine
Offer seminars and workshops on
health and personal development.
www.allaboutnaturalmedicine.com

Association of Master Herbalists
Herbalists trained in the tradition of
Dr John Christopher and Richard
Schulze.
www.associationofmasterherbalists.co.uk

CANCERactive
Holistic cancer information
www.canceractive.com

**College of Integrated Chinese
Medicine**
Acupuncture training college based in
Reading, which teaches an integrated
approach of Traditional Chinese
Medicine (TCM) and 5 Element
Acupuncture.
www.acupuncturecollege.org.uk

Cultured Probiotics
Suppliers of raw sauerkraut.
www.culturedprobiotics.co.uk

Greenpan
Non-stick frying pans that are not
toxic.
The Chandlery
Poole Road
Woking
Surrey GU21 6DY
Tel: 01483 255842
www.green-pan.co.uk

Helios Homeopathic Pharmacy
Manufacture and sell a huge range of
homeopathic medicines.
www.helios.co.uk

Hook and Son
Online mail order suppliers of organic,
raw, unpasteurised milk.
www.hookandson.co.uk

Make Yourself Better
A specific resource and information
site for the readers of this book. For
updates, newsletters and videos as well
as talks.
www.makeyourselfbetter.com

The Nutri Centre

A huge range of supplements and remedies and an extensive health and personal development bookshop.
7 Park Crescent
London W1B 1PF
Tel: 020 7436 5122
www.nutricentre.com

Philip Weeks Clinic

The author's clinic, providing personal consultations, individualised assessment and detoxification regimes. Probiotics, Nutrifood and herbal teas. Organised retreats are also available.
Wyeval House
42 Bridge Street
Hereford HR4 9DG
Tel: 01432 265565
www.philipweeks.co.uk

Planet Health

Biodegradable household cleaners as well as the Q silica skin range and sustainable manuka honey.
1 Tithe Barn
Barnsley Park
Barnsley
Gloucestershire GL7 5EG
Tel: 01285 741130
www.planethealth.com.au

UK Centre for Living Foods

Raw food retreats based on the teachings of Ann Wigmore. Run by Elaine Bruce in Ludlow, UK.
www.livingfoods.co.uk

Wholistic Research Company

Suppliers of juicers, rebounders, enema kits and so on.
www.wholisticresearch.com

Wild Fermentation

Information about how to prepare fermented foods.
www.wildfermentation.com

TESTS

Apart from York Test, all the other laboratories are a practitioner-only resource. To access a test you will need a referral by a qualified practitioner.

Acumen

A laboratory that will test for DNA adducts and mitochondrial function.
PO Box 129
Tiverton
Devon EX16 0AJ
Tel: 07707 877175
Email: acumenlab@hotmail.co.uk

Biolab Medical Unit

An excellent laboratory that I use to assess vitamin and mineral profiles, including red cell magnesium, and provides gut permeability testing and dysbiosis.
The Stone House
9 Weymouth Street
London W1W 6DB
Tel: 020 7636 5959/5905
www.biolab.co.uk

York Test Laboratories Ltd

They supply a finger prick test to determine whether you have an IgG food intolerance.
York Science Park
York YO10 5DQ
Tel: 01904 410410
www.yorktest.com

INDEX